THE 35-PLUS DIET FOR WOMEN

- is high in pro...
- provides calci...
- is high in fiber ... cholesterol
- is within the nutritional guidelines set down by the American Cancer Society and the American Heart Association

"HERE IS THE DIET THAT HAS HELPED HUNDREDS OF WOMEN LIKE YOU LOSE WEIGHT AND KEEP IT OFF. IT'S EXTREMELY SIMPLE TO FOLLOW AND VERY FLEXIBLE. *MORE THAN LIKELY, YOU HAVE EVERYTHING ON HAND TO BEGIN THIS DIET WITH YOUR VERY NEXT MEAL!*"—Jean Spodnik

"*THE 35-PLUS DIET FOR WOMEN* is not 'just another diet book.' Women in their 30s who have tried just about every crash diet on the market and just can't lose that 'middle-age spread' will be delighted to know that help is on the way."

—*Star Beacon*

JEAN PERRY SPODNIK, M.S.R.D., with over thirty years' experience as a nutritionist, is currently Lead Clinical Dietitian at the Kaiser Permanente Medical Offices in Cleveland, Ohio. She is also an instructor in the Department of Nutrition at Case Western Reserve University.

BARBARA GIBBONS is the author of "The Slim Gourmet" column, syndicated in more than 200 daily newspapers. Ms. Gibbons is the author of *The Slim Gourmet* cookbook, *Lean Cuisine* and *Diet Watcher's Cookbook*.

T H E
35
PLUS
DIET FOR
WOMEN

JEAN PERRY SPODNIK
and BARBARA GIBBONS

POCKET BOOKS

New York   London   Toronto   Sydney   Tokyo   Singapore

POCKET BOOKS, a division of Simon & Schuster Inc.
1230 Avenue of the Americas, New York, NY 10020

ISBN: 0-671-73213-7

First Pocket Books printing April 1988

15 14 13 12 11 10 9 8 7 6

POCKET and colophon are registered trademarks of
Simon & Schuster Inc.

KAISER PERMANENTE is a registered service mark
of Kaiser Foundation Health Plan, Inc.

Cover design by Mike Stromberg

Printed in the U.S.A.

*This book is dedicated in
the memory of my mentors:*

Clara Perry, my mother
Professor Helen A. Hunscher, Ph.D, R.D.
Professor Frances E. Fisher, M.S., R.D.

—Jean Perry Spodnik
Pepper Pike, Ohio
August 1986

Contents

I The 35-Plus Diet for Women

Before starting a diet, check with your doctor to be sure it is appropriate for you to go on a diet and that the diet you have selected is suitable for you.

While following the diet, if you experience any unexpected or unusual reactions or symptoms, consult your doctor promptly.

The case histories in this book are based on actual situations, but in some instances the cases are composites, and in all instances the names and identifying details about each person have been changed.

Introduction

Like lots of people predestined by genes to fatten up on fewer calories, I've found myself preoccupied by weight control, first as a frustration and finally as a career.

From the tubbiest toddler on the block, I grew to be the fattest kid in the eighth grade at 208 pounds. I spent the next twenty years exploring all the diets that don't work. In my thirties—married and a mother—I finally found slimness. Quite simply, I taught myself how to cook all over again.

Accepting finally the fact that I couldn't eat like other people, I began editing out the unneeded calories that made favorite foods more fattening than they needed to be.

Losing Weight in the Kitchen

Lightening up on calories in the kitchen is accepted practice today, but it was quite unheard of when I began doing it. I had to invent an entire cuisine just for myself, a way of cooking that focuses on

lean protein foods and bulky vegetables to satisfy the appetite

lots of spices and herbs and flavor-rich ethnic ingredients to make healthy food taste good

the avoidance of empty-caloried fats, sugars, and starches.

I lost eighty pounds and managed to keep it off. Because my true goal was to lose ninety! (Frankly, it still is.) At 128 pounds I was on the low side of the charts for my 5-foot 6-inch height, but I was still short of the model-skinny slenderness idealized in the media. So, my "diet" became permanent by virtue of never reaching its objective.

However, since my food-lover's approach led me to the exploration of ever-more interesting and exotic ways of combining low calorie foods into interesting meals and menus, I felt no deprivation. And my new set of food choices—lean meats, poultry, seafood, fresh fruits and vegetables, whole grains, herbs and spices—became preferred.

In 1971, I "turned pro." A newspaper reporter, I began sharing my ideas—in print—with others who wanted to lose weight while enjoying food. The "Slim Gourmet" column I wrote for a local newspaper quickly became syndicated, ultimately to more than 200 newspapers. I wrote cookbooks and low calorie cooking features in national magazines.

As a newspaper columnist for fifteen years, with weight control as my main "beat," I've observed the flow of fads and fashions, the shift in diet focus from anti- to procarbohydrate. Dieters used to eat the hamburger and throw away the bread. Ten years later, by the middle eighties, the hamburger was being thrown away. The focus was on less meat and more potatoes, more breads and pastas and other starchy fare. Once shunned, they were now favored. The diet books on the best-seller list changed from high protein to high carb.

Readers Share Weight Problems

My three-times-weekly newspaper column puts me in touch with readers' weight problems, and the mail delivers fresh insight daily. Lately there's been a noticeable increase in what I call the eat-like-a-bird letters: complaints from people, usually women, who failed to lose weight despite ultrastrict calorie-counting. Such women fill doctor's offices—not to mention doctors' wallets—yet more often than not reap only dismissal of their complaints. It's easy to conclude that they are simply kidding themselves. Indeed, the dietetic journals often feature research demonstrating how inept dieters are at recalling what they had for lunch and breakfast.

This marked increase in mail from women with similar complaints seemed to be coming from women entering their prime—women in their midthirties and older who were experiencing similar frustrations with conventional weight-loss regimens. As a group, they tended to be rather well-informed about current thinking on nutrition, high in self-awareness, and conscientious about their weight. It didn't seem possible that all of them were deluding themselves when they reported that conventional diets just didn't work for them anymore.

It was at this point that I had a propitious meeting—in print—with Jean Perry Spodnik, the developer of the 35-Plus Diet.

In my ongoing watch for news of interest to my diet-conscious readers, I generally search several medical, health, and nutrition journals every month. That's how I came upon the article in the *Journal of the American Dietetic Association* that told about a dietician's experiments at the Kaiser Permanente Medical Center in Cleveland, relating to the problems women over thirty-five have losing weight on conventional diets. It talked about a revolutionary diet that was achieving unprecedented success.

The three-phase diet worked its magic by precisely manipulating the *balance* among the three food elements, proteins, carbohydrate, and fats, replacing simple carbohydrate foods—sugars and refined starches—with fiber-rich whole grains, fruits, and vegetables. The diet augments these foods with lean protein from meat, poultry, fish, and dairy products.

The intentionally nonsensational language of the medical journal masked the excitement that this diet was ultimately to cause.

For one thing, it flew in the face of the current pro-carbohydrate diet wisdom: that less meat and more potatoes is just what the doctor ordered. The spectacular success of dieters in Jean Spodnik's program indicated that less meat and more potatoes is NOT what the doctor should order. At least not for women who are overweight and over thirty-five!

While this diet was drastically different from the high protein fad diets of the sixties and seventies—dramatic and substantial differences we'll detail later—certain essential aspects of this diet explain why those diets were so popular. The reason high protein crash diets have always been popular is because they work—in the short run at least—and nothing succeeds like success. They work because they cause a dramatic loss of water weight in the beginning, and this is a significant morale booster.

However, they did not work in the long run, because ultimately, calories do count! Despite the fact that these high protein fad diets provided a temporary quick fix for the water-retention aspect of women's weight problems, most of them were too high in calories, fat, and animal fats in particular. Beyond that, they were woefully and often dangerously unbalanced, and uniquely dangerous to women over thirty-five. This was true for several reasons:

• The high protein fad diets often made no distinction among the various kinds of carbohydrate. To a woman practicing carbo-counting, there was little difference between chili beans and chocolate bars. In her zeal to control the intake of carbs, it was logical to avoid the complex carbohydrates along with the simple—the whole grains, fruits, and vegetables along with sugar cookies and soda pop. Constipation often accompanied these diets, but that was the least of the woes they could cause.

- High protein diets promoted high fat intake, which is related to increased cancer risk. And they promoted it among the very people most at risk: overweight women.
- The excessive intake of fat, especially cholesterol-laden animal fat, increases the risk of heart disease at the very age when women are beginning to lose the hormonal protection that makes them less susceptible than men.
- The often excessive and unbalanced meat intake promoted the loss of calcium from the bones—the actual washing away of bone tissue that would ultimately result in osteoporosis ("porous bones"). Tragically the person most attracted to dieting was the very person most at risk: the weight conscious woman age thirty-five-plus.

In the decade that followed the heyday of the best-selling high protein "doctor diets," dieticians made their voices heard, and the dangers of these unbalanced diets became so well publicized that their appeal languished.

How America Eats Is Changing

In the last ten years there have been a number of factors that worked in concert to make profound changes in the American way of eating.

In the past the subject of food and cooking was primarily the preserve of housewives on the one hand and professional chefs on the other. And health? That was the preserve of the medical professional. Who wanted to hear about ailments when they sat down at the dinner table!

But now things were changing: members of youthquake had grown up. Better educated, inquisitive, iconoclastic, a new generation of adult consumer-oriented activists was moving into the mainstream. And they brought with them their dislike of plastic foods, their distrust of food manufacturers, and their disinclination to hand over control of their health to doctors and drugs.

In the new era people were encouraged to take charge of their medical well-being by adopting life-style changes that would promote longevity. And everyone was urged to participate, men as well as women. Dinner was no longer disconnected from how you felt, what you weighed, how long and how well you were likely to live.

And dinner was no longer the exclusive charge of "housewives"—since there were fewer of them.

With the soaring divorce rate and delayed marriages, many men were forced to cook for themselves. With different attitudes and the breakdown of traditional roles, many men were cooking for their families, or for the fun of it, or with health concerns in mind (and more often, all of the above). The physical fitness boom was an integral part of these changes.

The Fitness Phenomenon

The weight control diets of the late seventies and early eighties reflected all these changes as well as the changing demographics. Whereas in the past the typical dieter was a woman approaching, in, or past midlife (only women worried about weight gain, and this was a problem related to getting older), the more recent food and diet focus was now on body-conscious young adults, male and female, who jogged and worked out, often at the posh upscale coed "fitness centers" that were replacing singles bars. The menus that became popular mirrored the nutritional needs and life-style of young, active men and women in their twenties. Red meat became a nutritional no-no, and pasta was king. Running shoes became status symbols, and marathon mania was the nation's latest sweaty excess. Laurel-crowned contenders were photographed downing plates of pasta—carbohydrate-loading—to pack in that extra energy to go the distance. A nation of headline readers got the message that starch was in.

Today, the first of a whole generation of bread-eating, pasta-loving females is beginning to push forty. Most of them do not run in marathons.

They are experiencing the thirty-five-plus weight gain double-whammy: metabolic slowdown calling for fewer calories and hormonal changes calling for tighter control of carbohydrate intake. While most of today's weight-loss diets control calories, they tend to be high in carbohydrates. *They fail to address the hormonal changes that make this group of women fail on such diets.*

All of these observations were on my mind when I read of Jean Perry Spodnik's exciting experiments. I tracked the dietician down at the Kaiser Permanente Medical Center in Cleveland and set up an interview.

An attractive, personable, and compassionate woman, Jean Perry Spodnik was at first somewhat bemused by all the fuss her landmark research was creating. Her main interest was to help the ever-increasing stream of women over thirty-five who just weren't getting anywhere with weight loss by conventional means.

What I learned in researching my newspaper article was that the dietician at Kaiser Permanente Medical Center had succeeded in developing a carbohydrate-controlled diet specifically for thirty-five-plus women that allayed appetite and resulted in dramatic weight loss. Moreover, she had demonstrated that her unique combination of food elements worked better than conventional low calorie diets. Her dieters lost *40 percent more weight* than a matched group of women on a conventional diet with the same number of calories.

Jean and I developed a quick rapport. I had been favorably impressed with her work in the professional journals. She had an equal admiration for my work with food and had been bringing my books and recipes to her patients' attention. We quickly agreed to work together in bringing this diet to a wider audience, with expanded menus and a complete cookbook section with recipes designed especially for the 35-Plus Diet. We agreed that in addition to providing the diet and the recipes, we wanted also to produce a book that spoke directly to the 35-Plus Woman about the metabolic and hormonal changes that are happening to her so she understands the problems she is having and the solutions.

After this introduction, I'll turn you over to Jean for an explanation of the diet and guidance through its phases. In the second half of the book, we'll meet again through my recipes, designed specifically to bring enjoyment to the 35-Plus Diet.

Barbara Gibbons
Verona, New Jersey
August 1986

1 35 and Over: Why Nothing Seems to Work Anymore

Deirdre Parker, one of my patients, has just turned forty. This puts her among America's first Yuppies. I'm sure she qualifies. She has a BMW, a PC, a VCR, an IRA, and a CPA—and twenty-five pounds of excess weight she can't seem to get rid of no matter what she does! And that includes state-of-the-art exercise equipment, a semivegetarian diet, and spa cuisine.

Cool and self-assured depite the trace of annoyance that creased her brow, Deirdre was a financial adviser, and Job One was to inspire client confidence.

"I hate to fail at things, but this weight problem has me beat. I have a closetful of expensive custom-tailored suits, and this is the only one that still fits!" It was flawlessly tailored soft rose tweed, set off with a pink silk shirt and a rope of pearls that were almost certainly real.

Deirdre approached her weight problem the same way she approached everything else in her life—as a challenge to be met. First there was research, books and articles to read. An intelligent, informed consumer and nobody's fool, Deirdre easily and quickly separated fad from fact. So she had decided on a diet devised from contemporary nutrition wisdom: less protein and fat, and more "complex carbohydrates." In other words, less meat and more potatoes. Or in Deirdre's case, less pâté and more pasta salad.

But after two weeks of dieting, Deirdre was still at ground zero, having regained in the second week the single pound she lost in the first.

Disappointed but not yet defeated, she focused on calorie counts. "I figured it was like a company that didn't have a tight rein on costs. Slippage was somewhere, and I was determined to plug up the leaks." She ordered the comprehensive *Composition of Foods, Handbook 8* from the Government Printing Office and began meticulous calorie bookkeeping of her daily diet on a spread sheet she set up on her computer. She used a postage scale to weigh portions.

At the end of another month, Deirdre had lost three pounds on what she knew to be a 1,200-calorie nutritionally balanced diet. On her fortieth birthday Deirdre celebrated with two scoops of Häagen-Dazs chocolate ice cream and gained it all back.

Deirdre's experience typifies the irksome refusal of the human body to conform and perform according to predictable formulas. There's something so official and numerical about calorie guides that it's easy to slip into the expectation that our bodies will act like credit cards or bank accounts.

"I went on a semistarvation diet for one week and the scale in the doctor's office showed a two pound weight gain. He didn't believe me and accused me of cheating."

Such stories are nearly universal. The women who show up in doctors' offices tend to share a common experience: an unremitting pileup of pounds that begins in midthirties and escalates into midlife no matter what deprivations are undertaken to counteract it. And the doctors (usually male) don't believe them.

If you're a woman approaching or well into midlife, chances are you're battling weight gain. Suddenly (in some cases, or insidiously in others) the pounds pile up. What makes it all the more frustrating is that there's no dearth of diet advice. Yet the diets that seem to work for others—for your daughters, for the twenty-five-year-olds in the office, for the man in your life—just don't work for you.

You may have gone on a diet with your husband, perhaps even made a contest out of it, and in a short time he's lost the weight he wanted to lose—while you're still struggling with the first three pounds. You may have discovered that your first trip abroad—all that French and Italian food—put ten pounds on you and a month of dieting back home has lowered your spirits, but not your weight. As we leave youth behind, more and more we find that we just can't lose weight as easily as we once did. What has been a cinch becomes a challenge, then a chore, and finally an insurmountable obstacle. We may lose half a pound and then put it back on immediately—for no apparent reason.

I have been a registered dietician for thirty years and have heard these stories repeatedly from my women patients. I understand the women who come to me about weight problems at the Kaiser Permanente Medical Center in Cleveland, and I know they're telling the truth. I understand their frustration, particularly with those male diet doctors who dismiss them as cheaters and gluttons.

I have my own firsthand insight into how hormones can work mischief with the metabolism. The surgical removal of my ovaries—a hysterectomy—plunged me suddenly and prematurely into menopause. As the scale climbed incomprehensibly, I could understand the feelings of helplessness my patients were talking about.

My feelings of helplessness were all the more profound because I had all the answers—but the answers didn't work. I knew how to count calories, but somehow counting calories didn't seem to count anymore. Nor did any of the other remedies: more exercise, less salt, more meals, smaller servings. I found myself standing on the scale and cursing it as if it were a living breathing thing, just as I had seen so many of my patients do in helpless frustration after a week of white-knuckled table-pushing yielded no loss whatsoever.

I didn't know what was happening, but I did have an idea, and I went after federal funding to test a theory I had. The shared experience of my over-thirty-five Kaiser Permanente dieters seemed to suggest that as women proceed into their prime, there are subtle but profound changes in metabolism that are out of sync with today's eating fashions.

The Prime-of-Life Water Problem

The core of the problem seems to be secret water retention, leading to a fat and fluid buildup that signals its presence mainly on the scales. Or in swollen hands and feet. Take the case of Alice, a recent divorcee.

Alice had intended to make a grand gesture: pulling the wedding ring off her finger and tossing it at her ex's feet, just as he had tossed away her and their twenty-three-year marriage. But the actual scene was almost comic: The gold band refused to come off—it was wedged between two ridges of puffy translucent flesh. Alice's fingers were always like that at night. If I ever get a chance to replay this scene, Alice told herself grimly, I'll do it in the morning. She still had her sense of humor.

Scientific studies have shown that, after thirty-five, women are plagued with a special kind of fluid retention. My research revealed that this wasn't the ordinary pound or two you add temporarily during a heat wave or after an excessively salty meal.

I'm not talking about preperiod puffiness, either. Significant premenstrual bloat usually starts in our thirties and is much worse for some than for others. Each month, before our periods begin, our bodies produce fewer hormones, and this deficiency will cause fluid retention and premenstrual tension. (It also raises insulin levels, by the way, which in turn causes hunger, particularly the craving for sweets that many of us experience right before our periods are due. But that's another story we'll get into later.)

I'm talking here about a phenomenon common to many

women in their thirties, forties, and fifties. Conventional calorie counting is no match for the problem. Sodium-restriction diets fail to work in the long run. Moreover, the current switch to high carb diets, low in meat, appears to be all wrong for many midlife women. However healthy they are for men and for younger women, for women in midlife they can contribute to water retention and bloat.

After thirty-five, as we move closer to what the doctors call premenopause, we have a diminishing production of all female hormones with each menstrual cycle. And the hormone production does not increase after the period is over, as it did when we were younger.

The human body is composed of a significant amount of water. How is the water distributed in our bodies? Ideally, about half of it is inside the cells, and the rest of it is outside, between the cells and in the blood.

Here again, however, men and women differ. And fat people and thin people differ. Lean individuals with lots of muscles and little fat tend to have more of their body water within the cells. Women, especially fat women, tend to have more water between the cells.

When we retain water, it flows from the blood to the spaces between the cells, and the result is puffiness: thickened waistlines and bloated bellies. For some, but not all, it may also cause more obvious swelling in the legs and arms, especially the hands.

What's happening?

Our kidneys are performing an overenthusiastic favor for our blood. Since the blood must have sodium (salt) to do its job, the kidneys hold on to sodium so that blood is assured of an adequate supply. However, in the case of the bloated woman, the kidneys are storing too much sodium. And the body responds by matching the oversupply of sodium with an overbalance of water between the cells. The result? You can't get your shoes on or your ring off. Belts and blouses may not fit anymore, either!

Get rid of the extra sodium your body is retaining, and you'll get rid of the excess fluid between the cells.

The logical remedy, you would think, is to go on a low sodium diet and attempt to eliminate visible salt from your diet. I say visible, because you can't eliminate the natural sodium in the food itself. For a low sodium diet to help this kind of water retention, you would have to reduce sodium intake to less than one gram. That's tough, believe me! It's one of the most unpalatable diets there is—and very difficult to manage, requiring all sorts of special products. Since sodium is vital to life, such a diet is not without dangers also. You'd need to be under a doctor's care if you were going to restrict your sodium intake that drastically.

You might also get your physician to prescribe a diuretic (water pill). But prolonged use of diuretics without strict supervision may cause kidney damage. (Did you know that some reducing pills purchased over the counter actually contain a diuretic: ammonium chloride? You should be wary of using such preparations without medical advice.)

Neither diuretics nor salt-free diets have proved to be much help with the kind of weight problem that plagues the thirty-five-plus woman.

A Quick Fix for Water Weight

However, there is a kind of diet that does provide a quick fix for water weight problems. Promoters of fad diets have known about it for years. I call it the "Get Rich Quick Diet" because it has helped line the pockets and fund the retirement accounts of lots of diet promoters—without really solving the weight problems. Women may lose ten or fifteen pounds (more accurately, pints) very quickly and rave to their friends about this kind of diet, thereby helping to promote sign-ups or sales. But the minute they go off the diet, the body compensates and quickly brings its store of water back to prediet levels.

It is the high protein fad diet, and variations on it move in and out of fashion like shoulder pads and skirt lengths. It's been around for more than a hundred years in one form or another. And it's not only hucksters who employ this kind of diet. Variations of it are also used by concerned and ethical physicians who are trying desperately to help their overweight patients slim down. They use it because they know it works. But they don't know why. Or even with whom. They couldn't quite account for its effectiveness because until now there was no scientific evidence to back it up. But experience (what the medical community calls "anecdotal evidence") taught them that it worked more often than other methods. Why did it work? Chances are, most of their patients were 35-Plus Women. The majority of dieters have always been women over thirty-five, the patients most likely to show dramatic weight losses on a short-term high protein low carbohydrate regimen.

The Ketogenic Diet Extreme

Most of the fad diets over the years have delivered initial quick water-weight loss by taking the high protein diet to an extreme—by putting the dieter into ketosis.

Ketosis is a complication of starvation, a condition that results from the incomplete combustion of fatty acids. It's an outcome of following a diet with too little food, or more specifically, too few carbohydrates. While ketosis is a condition most would normally want to avoid, some of the high protein fad diets purposely brought it about by recommending diets devoid of adequate carbohydrate. Foods are composed primarily of protein, fat, and/or carbohydrate in various combinations. By manipulating the diet to short-

change basic carbohydrate needs—by minimizing not only
sugars and starches but also fruit, grains, legumes, and
vegetables—the body could be thrown into ketosis even
though caloric intake in the form of protein and fat was
adequate.

But ketosis is dangerous. The Council on Foods and Nutrition published a statement criticizing these high protein,
high-fat diets. They warned of metabolic problems that
could develop as a result. These problems are related to the
excessive excretory demands of the high protein intake and
included the possibility of life-threatening electrolyte im-
balance. With most of these diets, the dieter is directed to
stay on them only for a very short time (usually no more
than two weeks), because the authors are aware of their
harmful effects.

In fact, many of these high protein diets allow unlimited
amounts of high fat foods and ultimately don't result in
weight loss at all. If your energy (calorie) intake is greater
than your output (calorie needs), there is no way that you
can lose weight. You may lose excessive water, but not actual fat. And once you stop dieting, the water comes back.

The hormonal mischief that causes women to suffer fluid
retention is only one of the factors that makes weight loss a
bigger challenge for women than for men. The average
woman is programmed from puberty onward to store more
fat than her male counterpart does.

Female Metabolism

Let me tell you about one of my patients, Maggie. When
I first met her, she was visibly shaking with outrage—over
a word. The word was "obese."

That's what Maggie's doctor had written down on her

medical record. She had come to see him about her tiredness. When he left her alone in the examining room, Maggie tentatively tipped open the folder to see what he had written. And there was that word.

"What an awful word," Maggie wailed. Her doctor had referred her to me. I had the feeling that the text of her medical record was going to take precedence over losing weight. If I could have reclassified her as "big-boned" or even "substantially proportioned," she might have gone home in peace. But "obese"?

Having gained thirty-five pounds since college, Maggie would have grudgingly owned up to being perhaps a bit "overweight." But "obese" brought to mind "circus fat ladies, forgodsakes!"

But overweight and obese are not the same.

Obesity is the medical term for excessive fatness. To take Maggie's circus example, the strong man is "overweight." With his mantle of muscle, he weighs more than the average man of his height—even though he is actually underfat. But the circus fat lady (and Maggie, too, but I'm not going to tell her) are "overfat." In a word, obese.

It's probably safe to conclude that any woman who is thirty or more pounds heavier than the average woman of the same height is obese.

Why is it that the prime of life is marred for so many women by a relentless battle with the scale? Why is it that, for many of us, maturity brings obesity? The answer lies in our basic hormonal and metabolic makeup.

Metabolic Mischief

"My metabolism is low."

That's not simply an excuse used by lazy gluttons to explain away excess pounds. It is *the* reason why some people —especially women approaching midlife—start turning food into fat instead of fuel. Coupled with increased water retention, it spells double trouble for women over thirty-five.

But why is your metabolism low? Why now and not before? Why you and not him? Why do you feel like the fat lady married to the strong man? Too much food for you is never enough for him.

What is metabolism? *Metabolism* is a general term used to cover all the chemical changes that go on in the tissues of the body.

The "basal metabolic rate"—your BMR—represents the irreducible minimum of energy required to keep up the life processes, the internal work of the body. It is usually defined as the minimum amount of energy required by the body—the absolute least you would need when lying at rest in a comfortable environment, neither too hot nor too cold, completely relaxed, twelve to fifteen hours after the last meal. (Even digestion takes some energy.) You say that if you hadn't eaten for fifteen hours, you'd be anything but relaxed? Well, this is the theoretical "bottom line" that helps measure your basic energy needs.

The energy used to fuel the body can be measured: another term for a measure of energy is calorie.

Unfortunately for the fat lady, pound for pound it takes *fewer* calories to maintain her weight than it does for the strongman to maintain his, because fat takes very little energy to maintain.

Studies have shown that grossly obese persons tend to be relatively inactive. While the movements they do make are expensive in calories, they move so much less than persons of average weight that their stores of excess fat run little risk of being diminished.

But what many people do not realize is that muscles are *never* completely relaxed. Muscular tone is necessary even in sleep. Therefore, the muscular person will burn more calories, *even at rest,* than the obese person.

What does this mean for our extreme examples, the circus fat lady who is overfat and the circus strong man who is overmuscled? Simple. If they both tipped the scale at the same weight, the strong man could lose weight on a diet that would make the fat lady gain.

Hormones

You may be wondering why, in this era of equal opportunity, circuses still continue to feature strong *men* and fat *ladies*. To be sure, there are a lot more female body builders around today, but rarely do they achieve the spectacular musculature that their male counterparts do. Male hormones lead to the development of more muscles. Women's hormones, on the other hand, lead to the storage of fat. It's as simple as that.

Hormones dictate the laying down of fat on the female body in preparation for childbearing. From the very beginning of time, female physiology has been geared toward storing fuel in preparation for reproduction. When humans were hunters and gatherers, women had to be prepared not to gather while carrying their young. As soon as the young female of our species reaches puberty, her shape changes, and she begins to accumulate some fat around the hips. This accelerates during actual pregnancy. In the fourth to the sixth month even naturally slender women start to store fat around the derriere. I explain this to my young expectant mothers: Nature arranges things so that you can live off your own fat while the baby-to-be lives off your food.

Because of different body compositions in males and females, men have more active tissue than women. As little girls mature into young women, their hormones favor fat storage. As women mature and experience further hormonal changes, body composition continues to change: to less active tissue and more fat.

I use the term "active tissue" to describe men's muscles

How Active Are You?

In addition to your basal metabolic requirements, you must also take into account your activity level and how that affects the number of calories you need to maintain your weight. Here is a quick rule of thumb to see if you are as active as you think you are:

Very Light Activity Sitting most of the day: reading, talking, watching TV, studying. Only two hours or less spent walking or standing. This small amount of activity would take you only 30 percent above your basal metabolic needs. In other words, if your BMR is 1,000 calories, you would need only 1,300 calories to maintain your present weight, and anything above that would cause you to gain. Not very much, is it?

Light Exercise Sitting, typing, standing, laboratory work, some walking. This would be 50 percent above your BMR. It would take only 1,500 calories to maintain present weight.

Moderate Exercise Standing, walking, housework, gardening, carpentry, etc., little sitting. This would be 70 percent above your BMR or 1,700 calories to maintain present weight.

Strenuous Exercise Much of the time spent actively: standing, walking, skating, outdoor games, dancing, little sitting. This would be 100 percent above your BMR or 2,000 calories to maintain present weight.

Severe Exercise Laborers or professional athletes—tennis, swimming, basketball, football, running, heavy work. This could be 200 percent of your BMR or 3,000 calories to maintain present weight.

and "less active tissue" to describe fat. Actually, fat is just about inert. Think of it as simple *storage* of unused energy. Like anything tucked away unused and unneeded, it requires virtually no maintenance. The cost of its upkeep is very small compared to muscle.

Here's the metabolic bottom line:

Because of our different body composition—men with more muscles and women with more fat—women start off with a basal metabolic rate 10 percent lower than men.

So there you have it. Nature wants you to be fat!

Actually, when Mother Nature designed metabolisms, she didn't consider modern life-style, modern medicine, and your modern desire to live actively into your seventies and beyond. Nor did she imagine that mothers would want to look like their teenage daughters and that grandmothers would go on honeymoons.

But wait, it gets worse! Biologically, both men and women would reach their physical peak at age twenty-five. Metabolically speaking, after twenty-five it's downhill all the way. For both sexes. Our basal metabolic rate starts to decrease about 0.5 percent to 1 percent a year, varying from individual to individual. We usually don't notice this until we are in our thirties. By our forties, there's no doubt about it: We aren't burning calories the way we used to. The fact is, most women in this age group have a BMR of 1,000 calories or less.

2 The Challenge: Finding Out What Does Work

The challenge in developing a diet for the woman over thirty-five was to put together an eating plan that would restrict excess calories but still be appealing, satisfying, and nutritionally sound. At the same time, it had to get rid of the excess water and sodium in the body so that steady weight loss could take place.

Above all, it had to be a diet you could live with. A diet that leaves you hungry or edgy, that drains energy or compromises health, or one that's too demanding in what it requires or prohibits, will soon be abandoned.

A tall order!

The answer lay in food chemistry, in carefully calculating an exact balance of carbohydrate, fat, and protein in the diet. To achieve maximum results *it is essential that you follow the diet exactly*. While the 35-Plus Diet is very flexible within each food category, of necessity it is very rigid in its ratios.

This diet is *not* ketogenic. You will not experience the dry-mouth, bad-taste, bad-breath symptoms so familiar with ketogenic crash diets, nor the moodiness and lack of energy—that bone-tired weariness that starts to show up after the first week of a ketogenic diet. But it still lets the 35-Plus Woman get rid of water weight without the aid of drugs. And without eliminating salt. (The salt-free diet is one of the most difficult regimens a dietician has to deal with in therapy. Compliance is very low.)

Changing Your Body Chemistry

The 35-Plus Diet is set up in three phases. The first phase actually changes your body chemistry—alters your blood's chemical composition—so that you shed excess water. The second phase lets you continue to lose fat and excess water on a balanced-for-women diet that's easy to stay on. The third phase aims at keeping the weight off for good.

Phase One of the 35-Plus Diet is set up to bring you to the brink of ketosis, close to ketosis but not actually in it. In Phase One the composition of the diet is 27 percent carbohydrate, 40 percent protein, and 33 percent fat, a total of 900 calories. During this stage—which lasts one to two weeks—you can expect to lose 4 to 8 pounds.

Phase Two of the 35-Plus Diet is 37 percent carbohydrate, 34 percent protein, and 29 percent fat, a total of 950 calories. This ratio has proved to be ideal for the 35-Plus Woman dieter, and she can stay on it as long as she needs to. Despite its low-calorie total, it's designed to be appetite satisfying, with lots of bulky fiber foods and lean protein. Unlike other reducing diets, it does not foster the frustrating water weight fluctuations that defeat women dieters.

Phase Three is a "soft landing" readjustment into living the rest of your life without gaining excessive water or fat. In the last phase you gradually increase the use of carbohydrate foods experimentally—with weekends off your diet or alternate days off—until you find your own safe balance.

Calories Count But You Don't Have to Count Them

On the 35-Plus Diet, calories *do* count. But you don't have to, if you follow the diet plan. The caloric level is set close to most women's basal metabolic rate after thirty-five: under 1,000 calories in a 24-hour period. You don't need to count grams of carbohydrate or protein either. If you follow the diet, you will be assured of keeping your calorie intake low enough to lose fat. And your protein, fat, and carbohydrate intake will be properly balanced.

The diet has a double objective: (1) to lose fat, and (2) to force the body to give up the excessive sodium naturally, so you lose water. Keep in mind that it is the excess sodium in the body that is holding the excess water, which in turn accounts for your water retention problems and failure to lose weight on conventional low-calorie diets.

Flushing Away Excess Water

The body normally uses carbohydrate for energy. When the diet is manipulated—when protein foods rather than carbohydrate foods are being used to supply energy—the protein breaks down into hydrogen, carbon, oxygen, and nitrogen.

This last element is particularly significant. When nitrogen leaves the body by way of the kidneys, it picks up and flushes out sodium from the plasma (and potassium as well —more about that later). The body immediately seeks to replenish sodium in the plasma by taking it from the sodium-laden water between the cells—eliminating the excess water in the process.

These are the principles this diet puts to work:

1. Carbohydrates yield no ketogenic bodies and are, in fact, 100 percent antiketogenic.
2. Protein yields 46 percent ketogenic bodies and is 54 percent antiketogenic.
3. Fats yield 90 percent ketogenic bodies and are 10 percent antiketogenic.

All this means is that carbohydrate foods, like sugar and starch, do not promote ketosis, while protein and fat do.

Phase One of the 35-Plus Diet brings you just to the brink of ketosis by using a ratio of 1 to 1 between ketogenic and antiketogenic elements—more protein, less carbohydrate. Protein is the key here. Although fat is also on the ketogenic side of the balance, it has more than double the calories of protein, so intake of fat must be limited on a weight-loss diet. You do want to lose fat as well as water!

This careful balance of these three food elements is the key to the success of the 35-Plus Diet. While complex carbohydrates have an essential role in the diet, carbohydrate in the form of sugar is another story.

Sugar, Insulin, and the Menstrual Cycle

The pernicious role of sugar in the adult woman's diet can hardly be overstressed. Sugar conspires with the interplay of women's hormones in ways that increase hunger and contribute to the laying down of fat and the retention of water between the cells.

You may have noticed an increase in sweet cravings just before your period. This is due to a drop in estrogen that precedes the menstrual cycle. This, in turn, kicks off a whole relay of powerful hormonal recalibrations and reactions that literally turn your body into a fat-making machine:

- The decrease in estrogen causes the pituitary gland to pump out a natural antidiuretic.
- That interferes with the body's ability to flush away salt and water—so you have water retention.
- At the same time the insulin level goes up.
- This causes hunger, particularly a craving for sweets.
- If you answer that craving with sugar and excess calories,

you add to your fat stores and intensify your fluid retention problems.

Even worse, giving in to a craving for sweets sets up a self-
perpetuating roller coaster ride for your blood sugar level:
Sugar, especially refined sugar (sucrose), is pure carbohydrate, absorbed into the bloodstream much more quickly
than any other food component. When sweet freaks and
sugar junkies talk about "mainlining" sugar, they don't
know how apt the metaphor is. After eating sweets, the
level of sugar in the blood skyrockets. The body answers
with a rush of insulin, sending blood sugar levels down
precipitously low and setting up another bout of nervous
shaky sweet-craving—until your next sugar "fix."

Many women with weight and water-retention problems
are on a constant sugar high. This is why many women who
understand the problems they are having come to view
sugar as *addictive*. It's not addictive in quite the same way
that drugs are addictive, but it may be hard to tell the difference when you're on the roller coaster and your moods
and energy levels peak and plummet along with your blood
sugar levels.

Happily, you can get off sugar pretty easily, simply by
manipulating the diet to keep your blood sugar levels on a
fairly smooth line, rather than up and down. *You may experience sugar withdrawal during the first twenty-four to
forty-eight hours of the diet.* But it will pass. The trick is to
prevent the craving for sweets by filling up on lean protein
and high-fiber foods. Lean protein foods (lean meat, fish,
poultry, low-fat cheeses) are more slowly digested than carbohydrates. Bulky foods that are naturally high in fiber
such as whole grains, vegetables, and fruits—even though
these contain natural fruit sugars—also slow down digestion. This promotes a flatter blood sugar response than the
roller coaster ride you've been experiencing.

In dealing with this problem, you need to remember that

it's not just the sweets you eat that can contribute to blood sugar bounce. What about the sweets you drink? Sugar-sweetened soda, coffee, and tea, for example. I've had patients who were doing twelve Cokes a day. Caffeine, usually found in all three, by itself lowers blood sugar levels, making sugar withdrawal even more precipitous. If you are having problems with sugar, you should avoid these drinks or switch to sugar-free, decaffeinated brands. You should be able to tolerate moderate caffeine use again after blood sugar levels have stabilized.

Understanding how this diet works also makes it clear why sugar rather than salt is the bloat-causing culprit for many 35-Plus Women with weight problems. It has been well established in nutrition that placing obese patients on a diet totally of carbohydrates—regardless of the amount of sodium (salt) in the diet—prevents the loss of excessive sodium and water in the urine. When the same patients are then put on a diet solely of protein and fat (a ketogenic diet), they lose the sodium and water in the urine—regardless of the amount of sodium in the diet.

All of this should make it clear why it's important to be diligent in avoiding refined sugar and sugar-containing foods while following the diet. Unless you are on a sodium-restricted diet prescribed by your physician, you should follow the latest American Heart Association guidelines on salt, which suggests that you not exceed the equivalent of one teaspoon per day.

Putting the 35-Plus Diet to the Test

Like Dr. Jekyll, I found my best first subject right in the mirror. It was a mirror I was starting to avoid since a hysterectomy had thrown me into "instant menopause."

Menopause marks the end of a woman's childbearing years but by no means the end of her vitality and sexuality.

While motherhood is an important and fulfilling role, it's not the only one. The end of the childbearing cycle, coming at a time when most women would no longer want children anyway, ought to be welcomed with the same eagerness that young girls show for the beginning of the childbearing cycle.

After the ovaries are removed and a woman no longer has periods, the hormonal output ceases abruptly, not in the natural, gradual manner that usually occurs over a two-decade cycle. The forces that conspire to put on weight and water can suddenly overwhelm a woman after such surgery. I put on twenty pounds in just a few months. And not twenty pounds I could hide, either. I was bloated, distorted, and downright miserable. I love my work, and I love dealing with people, but who's going to take diet advice from a dietician who looks like she needs to go on a diet? I remember thinking that I'd have to give up my practice and hide in the lab with a loose white lab coat for a uniform.

In my first week on the experimental diet I lost five pounds. It was hard not to be thrilled, even though I knew, better than anybody, that this was "water weight," and celebration would be premature. The important questions were whether I'd continue to lose weight and if it would *stay* off. It took another two months to lose the remaining pounds. It was tempting—in view of today's extremely lean role models—to continue on and attempt to be model-slim, but my common sense and my nutrition education told me otherwise. Unreasonable expectations are a major cause of diet failure.

With my own success, I began using the diet with some of my more discouraging cases, the women who'd lose four pounds one week and gain back five the next.

What a revelation! Every last one succeeded in shedding the pounds that heretofore had stuck to them like glue. For many of them it was their first success ever, despite years of struggle. As I began using the diet with more and more women, I knew I was on to something. What was needed now was proof that it worked better than conventional diets. Simply adding up the pounds or the people who lost weight was not enough. We needed a controlled study.

As I suspected, given the results of the first early trials, there was no lack of volunteers willing to try out any diet that even *hinted* it might solve the problems of midlife weight loss. But proper research techniques required that we have a control group for purposes of comparison. That meant that for every woman on this 35-Plus Diet, there had to be another woman—similar in age and weight—on a conventional low-calorie diet.

The research was conducted with twenty healthy women between the ages of forty and sixty who were twenty to fifty pounds overweight. Ten were put on the diet I had devised, the test diet, and the other ten served as controls. They were put on a conventional balanced weight reduction diet of the same number of calories: 950. The composition of the other diet, the conventional calorie-counting diet, was 50 percent carbohydrate, 20 percent protein, and 30 percent fat, in accordance with the Recommended Dietary Goals for the United States set by the Select Committee on Nutrition and Human Needs of the United States Senate in 1977.

The study lasted seven weeks. Here's what happened:

The women on the conventional control diet experienced weight fluctuations and a widely diverse range of results. Over the seven-week period they ranged from a *gain* of one and one-quarter pounds to a loss of nine and one-quarter pounds. The average weight loss for the conventional diet was three and six-tenths pounds.

Those on the 35-Plus Diet, on the other hand, experienced a steady decline in weight and lost between nine and sixteen pounds over the seven-week period. Their average loss was eleven pounds—three times the average loss of the control group.

The success of the diet over the long haul is perhaps even

more significant than these figures. Dieting statistics tell us
that only one person in twenty succeeds in reaching weight-
loss goals and keeping weight off. But since that first experiment, we've seen steadily mounting evidence that the
35-Plus Diet gives better and more consistent results than
virtually any other kind of diet for women in this age group.
As of this writing, it has been used with resounding success
with more than 7,000 women at Kaiser Permanente, and
better than 75 percent stick with it and succeed.

Findings from the original research, accepted and published in the *Journal of the American Dietetic Association*,
received worldwide attention in the medical community,
and practitioners from as far away as Israel and the Soviet
Union have asked for details of the diet, citing similar complaints from female patients in the over-thirty-five category.

Some Success Stories

Approximately one-third of the women I've worked with
in the program are between the ages of thirty and forty.
About half of my patients have been menopausal, postmenopausal, or have had hysterectomies. Their back-
grounds and experiences cover a wide range:

One patient was a secretary in her early thirties with a
sedentary office job who had experienced a gradual weight
gain over a period of years. She was wearing a size eighteen
when she started the 35-Plus Diet and went to a size ten in
eight months. As of this writing she's maintained her size-
ten figure for three years.

Another young woman had experienced a typical rapid
weight gain after her hysterectomy. Most of the added
pounds collected around her middle, and her fashionable
clothes no longer fit. She'd put on fifteen pounds in four
months, and took them off in three with the diet. The diet

was "a godsend," she said. "Now I don't have to buy my clothes at the half-size shop anymore!" She's maintained her weight loss for five years.

Another patient, I'll call her Jane, gained twenty pounds when she quit smoking. She is a nurse and keenly aware of the health risks of smoking *and* the problems associated with overweight. What Jane particularly liked about the 35-Plus Diet was the unlimited "chewables" offered by the unlimited vegetable list. She and her carrot sticks and broccoli buds got to be a joke around the office, but she lost the weight and now more than a year later is still a slender nonsmoker.

One sixty-year-old patient came to me with high cholesterol levels and thirty pounds of excess weight. With the diet she lost the weight and brought her cholesterol count down to a safe level at the same time. Another patient in her later sixties had both high cholesterol *and* high blood sugar. With the diet she lost twenty pounds and lowered both the cholesterol and blood sugar levels. Three years later her weight, her cholesterol, and blood sugar are still under control.

One petite mother of three had always had some weight problems but nothing had ever done much to solve them. In her midthirties her weight gain began to accelerate, and by the age of thirty-eight she was thirty pounds overweight. With the diet she finally brought her weight under control, losing thirty pounds in eight months.

Two patients of mine in their early thirties are very active physically. Each had put on only about ten unwanted pounds, but in both cases the gain was all in the midriff and all their exercising wouldn't budge it. The 35-Plus Diet got rid of the bulge—and the ten pounds—on both women.

Another nurse among my patients—I'll call her Mary—is in her late thirties. Mary changed from a physically demanding job on the night shift to a desk job—a change in

Some Features of the Diet:

Salt permitted. While the diet doesn't promote profligate use of the salt shaker, neither does it rule salt out. Some current findings on the subject of sodium question the wisdom of urging universal salt restriction to the general population, and I concur with that thinking. Potassium, found in fruits and vegetables, is the other part of the sodium seesaw, and this diet promotes abundant use of potassium-containing produce. (An important exception here is the individual who is part of that subgroup of sodium-sensitive people for whom salt restriction is important and effective in lowering blood pressure. Follow your physician's advice if you have a water retention problem or hypertension related to salt intake.)

Meat permittted, including beef and other favorite red meats. This diet does not follow the popular fashion, arbitrarily excluding beef or pork or other meats, frequently without any justification. (Some cuts of meat actually have less fat and calories than some poultry parts, and it is these ultralean sources of protein that are favored in the menus and recipes.)

Alcohol permitted, once you are into Phase Two. See Chapter 4 for details.

Controls hunger. Attacking, allaying, forestalling, and postponing hunger is a primary concern of any weight-loss diet, since the hungry dieter is soon an ex-dieter. This regimen works to prevent hunger on two fronts: at the table and away from it. At the table, by the liberal use of bulky, stomach-filling vegetables and other high fiber foods that prevent overeating at mealtime. To prevent nibbling between meals, the diet includes liberal amounts of slowly metabolized protein foods.

Deals with women's calcium needs. Many diets that have been popular are actually all wrong for the 35-Plus Woman because they exacerbate the tendency for maturing women to develop the calcium deficiencies that ultimately lead to osteoporosis, the loss of bone mass that makes the bones of elderly women brittle and breakable. Current research informs us that this is a condition that has its roots in the eating habits of several decades earlier. Unfortunately, the drive toward slenderness usually deprives women of the very nutrients they need most, and many popular weight-loss diets further the damage.

Changes metabolism. The 35-Plus Diet deals with the chemistry of fluid retention and blood sugar levels, and with another unseen and unrecognized enemy: the metabolic slowdown that results from excess fat. This is how weight gain not only becomes self-perpetuating but even picks up momentum as the weight problem remains unmanaged. This is how ten pounds turns into twenty and then fifty. The diet is designed to interrupt this vicious circle with a quick loss of water and fat. As the water flushes away and the fat melts, the metabolically inert burden disappears.

Nutritionally balanced. Unlike the high protein fad diets of the nineteen-sixties and nineteen-seventies featured in bestselling diet books, this diet provides the basis for a lifetime of healthy eating. Some of the differences:

The 35-Plus Diet is low in fat. No butter, margarine, oil, or fat-adding ingredients are included, and the protein foods used are lean: chicken, poultry, fish, only lean fat-trimmed meat. (The fad high protein diets of a decade ago called for large quantities of fatty steaks and hamburger.)

The 35-Plus Diet isn't overweight in protein. It allows about 80 grams per day; the nondieting typical American eats in excess of 100 grams. Some of the high protein fads put no limit on protein intake.

The 35-Plus Diet does allow unlimited amounts of complex carbohydrate vegetables—and fruit three times a day. Consequently, it's high in naturally occurring fiber. High protein fad diets of the past generally made little mention of fiber or fiber foods. In fact, they tended to discourage fiber food intake by not differentiating between complex carbohydrate high-fiber vegetables and simple carbohydrate foods like sugar and refined flour.

The 35-Plus Diet is enjoyable and easy to live with. It's versatile and flexible and fits into every life-style. It's equally adaptable whether you love to cook or hate it.

life-style that put twenty pounds on her in six months. She took them off in five with the diet, and as of this writing has kept them off for three years.

Pregnancy got the better of a patient I'll call Mrs. Grayson, who gained far too much weight while she was carrying her baby. I put her on the diet after the baby was born, and she lost thirty pounds in six months. She looks terrific. I told her to be sure to come in for a special prenatal regime the next time she gets pregnant. I figure it won't be too long.

3 The 35-Plus Diet

Here is the diet that has helped hundreds of women like you lose weight and keep it off. It's extremely simple to follow and very flexible. More than likely, you have everything on hand to begin this diet with your very next meal.

How the Diet Is Organized

The diet is organized around three "square" meals a day plus one any-time snack. If you generally eat your main meal at midday and a light supper in the evening, simply rearrange the diet schedule to make the second meal the main meal. The snack could be midmorning coffee break, or late afternoon pick-me-up or a healthy after-dinner "dessert."

At each of these meals you are directed to eat a number of units or *servings* of different kinds of foods: lean protein, grain, fruit, etc. *Servings* generally apply to 1 ounce or 1 unit (a peach, for example) or ½ cup. More on that later.

As we have seen, the diet has three phases, each subsequent phase allowing more food than the preceding one. Although the differences are not great, they are critical! For example: Phase One dinner calls for a healthy portion of protein plus unlimited light vegetables, but no bread or other starches in the main meal. In Phase Two, dinner is augmented by one starch serving—bread, for example, or potatoes, pasta, or rice.

Phase One is intended to jump-start your metabolism and turn it around into an energy-burning machine rather than one primed to store energy in the form of extra chins

or flabby thighs. Phase One permits only two servings of
starch food a day, one in the morning and one at lunch.

Phase One

You should stay on Phase One for one week. At the end
of seven days, you will probably be pleased to see a dramatic weight loss on the scale. You may lose five pounds or
more, depending on your body composition. Then you
should proceed to Phase Two. The amount of weight loss
varies with each individual. If you're a slow starter, you
should not be discouraged because the amount of weight
lost in the first week has little bearing on your ultimate
success. My observation of hundreds of women on this diet
discloses that some who lost the least weight at the beginning ultimately went on to achieve the most dramatic
weight loss in the end.

If at the end of the first week you have lost less than two
pounds, you should stay on Phase One for one more week
—*but in no case should you stay on Phase One more than
two weeks.*

Why is it important to limit Phase One to a maximum of
two weeks? Because of the danger of ketosis.

The ratio of carbohydrate to protein and fat in Phase One
is intended to bring the dieter to the *brink* of ketosis in
order to force the body to relinquish its store of excess water
between the cells. The body generally does this within a
week (although some particularly stubborn cases of water
retention may need a bit more time). Two weeks is the
maximum duration for a diet that's severely restricted in
necessary carbohydrates.

Phase Two

After the initial Phase One is over, the dieter moves on
to Phase Two. At first glance, the difference seems small—

one more slice of bread a day (or ½ cup of spaghetti)—but it is significant. The diet is carefully calibrated to provide just the right balance of lean protein and complex carbohydrate to foster the loss of fat and prevent a recurrence of waterlogging. For this reason, it's vital to follow the diet—exactly—in terms of portions and proportions of each type of food. Within those constraints, the diet is designed to provide maximum flexibility: You can interchange a wide variety of starch foods, enjoying corn on the cob one day and macaroni salad the next. But the diet will *not* work if you choose a second ear of corn instead of the broiled chicken, or if you decide to have less meat and more potatoes.

The ratio of protein to carbohydrate is important to keep the space between the cells squeezed dry of excess fluid. The amount of food you eat is important in retaining that ratio, as well as in keeping calories in check. Calories are important, but they have already been accounted for in the diet plan. If you eat more of a favorite food than the diet calls for—if you eat a food not permitted—you will sabotage your efforts both by overconsumption of calories and by destroying the protein–carbohydrate ratio that prevents water weight gain.

How long should you stay on Phase Two? For as long as you need to, until you have reached your desirable weight (we'll discuss weight goals, later). Unlike unbalanced high protein diets of the past, this is a safe, balanced diet that shortchanges only calories. So, as long as you have a ready supply of excess calories stored on your body, you can remain on Phase Two. This part of the diet is designed to draw on those fat reserves for energy, and to avoid replacing the lost fat by puffing up the spaces between the cells with water weight gain.

Phase Three

After you have reached the weight you want to be, you are then faced with the most demanding and difficult challenge of all: maintaining that weight loss for the rest of your life. This is where nineteen out of twenty diets fail. The 35-Plus Diet meets that challenge successfully with a third phase that will last the rest of your life.

In Phase Three, we add 3 servings (3 teaspoons) of fats —other than saturated animal fats—to the diet. Stay on the diet five days a week. On the other two days—the weekend, for example—you can indulge yourself within reason by enjoying modest portions of foods not permitted on the diet. Remain on Phase Three as long as your weight remains stable. If you regain more than five pounds, return to Phase Two and remain on it until the weight is lost.

After you have remained on Phase Three for more than two months without weight gain, you may add a third "day off" to your program, a midweek day for example, in which you might eat dinner out and enjoy a dessert. Or you might want to alternate days on and off your diet.

Again, if you regain more than five pounds, return to Phase Two and remain on it until the weight is lost and then return to Phase Three with only two days off.

Phase Three is intended to help you find a happy healthy level of food intake that can keep you well-fed for the rest of your life without regaining those unwanted extra pounds. It's important to understand and accept that you will never be able to go back to your old eating habits— unless you are willing to go back to the weight you used to be!

3 slices/oz

PHASE ONE   (One to two weeks, maximum)

Meal:	Breakfast	Lunch	Dinner	Anytime/Snack
		NUMBER OF SERVINGS		
Lean protein	1	3	6	—
Light vegetables	unlimited quantities, *at least 4 servings a day*			
Fruit	1	1	—	1
Skim milk/ yogurt	—	—	—	1
Grain/starch	1	1	none	none
Fats	none	none	none	none
Sugar	none	none	none	none
Alcohol	none	none	none	none
Calcium supplement	1	1	2*	—
Vit/Min supplement	—	—	1*	—

PHASE TWO   (Until goal weight is achieved)

Meal:	Breakfast	Lunch	Dinner	Anytime/Snack
		NUMBER OF SERVINGS		
Lean protein	1	3	6	—
Light vegetables	unlimited quantities, *at least 4 servings a day*			
Fruit	1	1	—	1
Skim milk/ yogurt	—	—	—	1
Grain/starch	1	1	1	—
Fats	none	none	none	none
Sugar	none	none	none	none
Alcohol	—	—	—	1 allowed
Calcium supplement	1	1	2*	—
Vit/Min supplement	—	—	1*	—

*Taken after dinner.

PHASE THREE   (5 days a week, to stabilize and
   maintain permanent weight loss)

Meal:	Breakfast	Lunch	Dinner	Anytime/Snack
		NUMBER OF SERVINGS		
Lean protein	1	3	6	—
Light vegetables	unlimited quantities, *at least 4 servings a day*			
Fruit	1	1	—	1
Skim milk/ yogurt	—	—	—	1
Grain/starch	1	1	1	—
Fats (mono & poly)	1	1	1	—
Sugar	none	none	none	none
Alcohol	—	—	—	1 allowed
Calcium supplement	1	1	2*	—
Vit/Min supplement	—	—	1*	—

*Taken after dinner.

Custom-Tailoring Your Menus

Three servings for lunch, six servings for dinner—does
that mean three Quarter Pounders and six pork chops?

To make the diet easy to follow and maximize the flexibility among foods that are interchangeable, we've used an
exchange system of units: small "servings" that can range
from 1 ounce of meat to ½ cup of vegetables, milk, or fruit.

Although calories count—absolutely—this exchange system relieves you of the need to count them! You can make your choices from the Food List in the next chapter. This allows you the most freedom to design a diet to suit your own likes and dislikes, your own life-style. Instead of a rigid one-size-fits-all diet—one that pinches and gaps and seems better suited to someone else—the 35-Plus Diet lets *you* custom-tailor menus and meal plans that meet your needs.

For example, the fruit and dairy foods under Anytime/Snack can be used anytime during the day—midmorning coffee break, say, or late afternoon energizer. Or the foods and drinks listed could be added to regular meals. The fruit could be added to dinner, as dessert. The milk could be utilized in breakfast cereal or throughout the day in coffee. The one alcoholic beverage allowed in Phase Two could be light beer with lunch or dry wine with dinner or a predinner cocktail or after-dinner brandy—pick one! It is also permissible to borrow 1 ounce of protein from dinner—a thick slice of low-fat diet cheese, for example—and have that as part of a midmorning or midafternoon snack.

A Diet for Men

Well, it needs some adaptation. This one is about 1,500 calories to accommodate differences in the male metabolism. If your man does physical labor or a lot of exercise, he may add additional servings of starch and fruit.

One feature of the Men's Diet is the addition of four servings of unsaturated fat. These include polyunsaturated margarine and vegetable oils such as corn and safflower oil, and monounsaturated fat such as olive oil. *I strongly urge that only unsaturated fats be used in the men's diet and that additional animal fat in the form of butter and cream be avoided.*

MEN'S DIET (Approximately 1,500+ calories)

Meal:	Breakfast	Lunch	Dinner	Anytime/Snack
		NUMBER OF SERVINGS		
Lean protein	1	3	6	1
Light vegetables	unlimited quantities, *at least 4 servings a day*			
Fruit	1	1	1	1
Skim milk/ yogurt	—	—	—	1
Grain/starch	2	2	2	1
Fats (unsaturated)	1	1	2	none
Sugar	none	none	none	none
Alcohol	none	none	none	1
Vit/Min supplement	—	—	—	1

4 The 35-Plus Diet Food Lists

LEAN PROTEIN FOOD LIST

Lean Meat	*One serving equals 1 ounce (cooked).*

Beef:
- bottom round roast or steak
- corned beef round
- cube steak
- eye round roast
- flank steak
- hamburger, diet lean
- lean beef stew meat
- minute steak
- round roast
- sirloin
- tenderloin
- top round steak

Veal: most cuts

Lamb: leg, leg steaks, loin chops, sirloin, fat-trimmed ground

Pork:
- center-cut fresh or cured ham
- pork tenderloin

Organ meats: liver (high cholesterol), limit to one 3-ounce serving per month)

Poultry: remove skin before or after cooking
- young frying chickens
- Cornish hens
- guinea hens
- pheasant
- young turkey

Lunch meats:
- most chicken and turkey alternatives
- light and deli-lean lunch meats 95 percent to 98 percent fat free

Game: venison, most game except waterfowl

LEAN PROTEIN FOOD LIST, *continued*

Medium Fat Meat
   Allowed no more than 3 times weekly. Trim carefully.

Beef:	chuck, shoulder, rump
Veal:	breast
Lamb:	arm chops, rib, loin
Pork:	Boston butt, picnic, shoulder

Avoid These High-Fat Cuts of Meat:

Beef:	rib steak, rib roast
	brisket
	corned beef brisket (corned beef round is
	permitted)
	regular hamburger
	porterhouse, T-bone steak
	Boston strip steak, club,
	plate, skirt
Lamb:	breast of lamb
Pork:	spareribs
	sausage
	ground pork
Poultry:	capon, duck, goose, waterfowl
Lunch meat:	regular wieners and hotdogs,
	salami, pastrami, veal loaf,
	most regular lunch meats

Fish and Shellfish
   One serving equals 1 ounce, cooked, without bones, skin, or shells.

Fish:	fresh and frozen: all varieties permitted
Shellfish:	raw, steamed, boiled, broiled, or baked
	clams
	crabs
	crayfish
	mussels
	oysters
	scallops

LEAN PROTEIN FOOD LIST, *continued*

Avoid: commercial breaded and fried fish
                 breaded and fried shellfish

       Fish and
       shellfish,
       canned: tuna packed in water or brine
                 salmon
                 crabmeat

           Fish,
       smoked: whitefish, salmon, kippers, sable, sturgeon,
                 mackerel, etc.

           Fish,
pickled, cured: salmon (lox)

Limit: no more than one 3-ounce serving per week
                 sardines in tomato sauce
                 sardines
                 shrimp
                 lobster

Avoid: herring in cream sauce
                 herring in sweet wine
                 sardines in oil
                 tuna packed in oil

DAIRY FOODS LIST

Cheese	*One serving equals:*
cottage cheese, low-fat (1 percent or less)	⅓ cup
fresh farmer's cheese (dry or pot cheese)	⅓ cup
light or diet processed cheese	1 ounce
mozzarella, skim light and part skim	1 ounce
Avoid: all full fat cheeses	

DAIRY FOODS LIST, *continued*

Eggs and Egg Substitutes

> egg whites (1 serving equals 2 whites)
> cholesterol-free substitutes (1 serving equals
> ¼ cup or the equivalent of one whole egg)
> whole eggs (1 serving equals 1 large)

Limit: egg yolks and whole eggs (high in cholesterol) limit to
2 per week

Skim Milk and Yogurt		*One serving equals:*
Milk:	skim, fresh	8 ounces
	skim, reconstituted	8 ounces
	skim, dry nonfat milk solids	4 tablespoons
	low-fat, 99 percent fat-free (1 percent fat)	8 ounces
	milkshake mix, low-calorie sweetener	1 packet
	cocoa mix, low-calorie sweetener	1 packet
	buttermilk	8 ounces
Avoid:	chocolate and other sugar-sweetened milk drinks	
	cream	
	half and half	
	low-fat milk with 2 percent fat or more	
	nondairy creamers (dry, frozen, liquid)	
	whole milk	
Yogurt:	plain skim milk yogurt	¾ cup
	plain low-fat yogurt	¾ cup
Avoid:	whole milk yogurt	
	fruit yogurt sweetened with sugar or fructose	

UNLIMITED VEGETABLES LIST

One serving equals ½ cup, cooked, or 1 cup, raw.

artichokes
asparagus
bamboo shoots
bean sprouts
beet greens
beets
broccoli
Brussels sprouts
cabbage
carrots
cauliflower
celery
chard
chicory
Chinese cabbage
collard greens
cucumber
dandelion greens
eggplant
endive
escarole
fennel
kohlrabi
leeks
lettuce

mixed vegetable juice
 (limit 1 cup)
mushrooms
mustard greens
okra
onions
peppers
pickles (dill, sour, or unsweetened)
radishes
romaine
rutabagas
sauerkraut
scallions
spinach
summer squash: yellow, crook-
 neck, pattypan, spaghetti,
 scalloped
string beans (green or wax)
tomato juice (limit to 1 cup)
tomatoes (limit to 1 medium)
turnip
turnip greens
watercress
zucchini

GRAIN/STARCH LIST

Bread   *One serving equals:*

bagels	½ regular
bread sticks	2 (8-inch)
bread crumbs	3 tablespoons
cracked wheat	1 slice
crispbread (high fiber)	2 pieces
English muffin	½ small
frankfurter bun	½ small

GRAIN/STARCH LIST, *continued*

Bread		*One serving equals:*
	French	1 slice
	hamburger bun	½ small
	"light" calorie-reduced	2 slices
	high fiber	2 slices
	Italian	1 slice
	pita pocket	1 ounce small
	protein enriched	1 slice
	raisin bread	1 slice
	roll, plain	1 half small
	rye, pumpernickel	1 slice
	tortilla, corn	1 (6-inch)
	tortilla, wheat	½ (8-inch)
	white	1 slice
	whole wheat	1 slice
Avoid:	biscuits	
	cake	
	coffee cake	
	cookies	
	corn muffins	
	cornbread	
	croissants	
	Danish pastry	
	doughnuts	
	fried croutons	
	French toast	
	pancakes	
	sweet rolls	
	waffles	

Crackers		
	arrowroot	3
	graham	2 (2¼-inch squares)
	matzo	1 (6-inch diameter)
	melba toast	4 (2¾ inch)
	oyster crackers	20

GRAIN/STARCH LIST, *continued*

Crackers		*One serving equals:*
	pretzel sticks	25 (3-inch)
	rye or wheat wafers	3 (2 x 3½ inch)
	saltines	6 (2½ inch squares)
	soda crackers	4 (2½ inch squares)
Avoid:	rich crackers	
	potato chips	
	corn chips	
	fried snack chips	

Starchy Vegetables, Cooked		
	acorn or hubbard squash	½ cup
	butternut squash, mashed	½ cup
	other winter squashes	½ cup
	beans, canned in sauce	¼ cup
	beans, dried, cooked	½ cup
	corn, kernels	⅓ cup
	corn on the cob	1 small
	hominy	½ cup
	lima beans, fresh	½ cup
	lima beans, dried, cooked	½ cup
	lentils, dried, cooked	½ cup
	mixed vegetables	½ cup
	parsnips	½ cup
	peas, green	½ cup
	peas, dried, cooked	½ cup
	potato baked with skin	1 small
	potato, cooked and mashed	½ cup
	pumpkin, plain	¾ cup
	yam or sweet potato, plain	¼ cup
Avoid:	French fries	
	sugary glazed yams, squash	
	sweet baked beans	

GRAIN/STARCH LIST, *continued*

Pasta		*One serving equals:*
	whole wheat	½ cup cooked
	protein-enriched	½ cup cooked
	egg noodles	½ cup cooked
Avoid:	fried chow mein noodles	

Cereal		
	oatmeal, cooked, plain	½ cup
	grits, cooked, plain	½ cup
	most cooked cereals	½ cup
	granola	¼ cup
	Fiber One	½ cup
	bran flakes, 100 percent	½ cup
	Cheerios	¾ cup
	corn flakes, wheat flakes	¾ cup
	puffed wheat, corn or oats	1 cup
	Special K	1 cup
	most ready-to-eat cereals	¾ cup
Avoid:	sugar-coated cereals	

Grains		
	barley, cooked	½ cup
	bulger, cracked wheat, cooked	½ cup
	couscous, steamed	½ cup
	popcorn, air-popped, no butter or oil	3 cups
	rice, brown cooked	½ cup
	rice, white cooked	½ cup
	rice, wild cooked	½ cup
Avoid:	sweet baked beans	
	fried rice	
	packaged or prepared rice, pasta, potato, couscous or other grain convenience mixes with added fat	

FRUITS LIST

Fresh, frozen, or canned in water or unsweetened juice. May be sweetened with sugar substitute if desired.

	One serving equals:
apple juice	⅓ cup
apples	1 small
applesauce (sugar free)	½ cup
apricot halves	½ cup
apricot nectar	⅓ cup
apricots (dried)	4 halves
apricots (fresh)	2 medium
banana	½ small
blackberries	½ cup
blueberries	½ cup
boysenberries	1 cup
cherries	10
cider	⅓ cup
cranberry juice	¼ cup
dates	2
figs (dried)	1 small
figs (fresh)	1 large
fruit cocktail	½ cup
fruit punch	¼ cup
gooseberries	⅔ cup
grape juice	¼ cup
grapefruit (fresh)	½ medium
grapefruit (juice)	½ cup
grapefruit sections	¾ cup
grapes	12 medium
Kiwi fruit	1 large or 2 small
loganberries	½ cup
mango	½ small
melon—watermelon	½ slice (1 cup)
melon—cantaloupe	¼ small
melon—honeydew	⅛ small
nectar (apricot, peach, pear)	⅓ cup

FRUITS LIST, *continued*

	One serving equals:
nectarine	1 small
orange	1 small
orange juice	½ cup
orange sections	½ cup
papaya	⅓ medium
peach (fresh or canned)	1 medium
pear (fresh or canned)	1 medium
persimmon	1 small
pineapple (canned)	1 large slice
pineapple (fresh)	½ cup
pineapple juice	⅓ cup
plums	2 medium
pomegranate (seeds)	¾ medium
prune juice	¼ cup
prunes	2 medium
raisins	2 tablespoons
raspberries	½ cup
rhubarb (no sugar)	¾ cup
strawberries	1 cup
tangerine	1 large or 2 small

FATS LIST

These foods and ingredients may be used only as directed in the recipes, and in Phase Three, and as directed in the Men's Diet.

Unsaturated Fats	*One serving equals:*
avocado	½ cup
cooking oil (corn, olive, safflower, sunflower, etc.)	1 teaspoon
margarine ("lite," diet or whipped)	2 teaspoons
margarine (soft or stick—first ingredient should be liquid oil)	1 teaspoon
mayonnaise	2 teaspoons

FATS LIST, *continued*

Unsaturated Fats	*One serving equals:*
mayonnaise (light or calorie-reduced)	1 tablespoon
nut butters, tahini	1 tablespoon
nuts and peanuts, dry-roasted or oil-roasted	½ ounce
peanut butter (all-natural)	1 tablespoon
salad dressings (light low-fat, calorie reduced)	2 tablespoons
salad dressings (bottled oil & vinegar type)	4 teaspoons
salad dressings (regular, bottled, mayonnaise-type)	1 tablespoon
seeds (pumpkin or squash kernels, sunflower seed kernels)	½ ounce
sour dressing, nondairy	3 tablespoons
wheat germ oil	1 teaspoon

Saturated Fats	
bacon (crisp)	1 ounce
bacon fat	1 teaspoon
butter	1 teaspoon
chocolate, unsweetened baking	1 ounce
coconut (shredded)	1 ounce
coconut cream, unsweetened	3 tablespoons
cream (half and half, 10 percent butterfat)	2 tablespoons
cream (heavy, 18 percent butterfat)	1 tablespoon
cream (sour)	2 tablespoons
cream cheese (regular and whipped)	2 tablespoons
cream cheese spreads	2 tablespoons
cream substitute (liquid or dry—Cremora or Coffee Rich)	2 tablespoons

FATS LIST, *continued*

Saturated Fats	*One serving equals:*
cream, whipped heavy (unsweetened)	2 tablespoons
lard	1 teaspoon
margarines from hydrogenated fats (regular stick)	1 teaspoon
salt pork	½ ounce
sausage, regular pork breakfast bulk or links	1 ounce
sauces and gravies, made with butter, fat or oil	⅓ cup

Avoid These Foods

biscuits
cake
candy
chow mein noodles
cookies
corn muffins
cornbread
croissants
doughnuts
frozen custard
frozen tofu desserts
frozen yogurt
fruit-flavored yogurt with sugar
honey
ice cream
ice milk
jam, jellies, and preserves
Jell-O and gelatin desserts, sugar-sweetened
lemon ice, other sugar-sweetened fruit ices
molasses
muffins
pancakes
pies
potatoes, French fried

pudding and dessert mixes, sugar-sweetened
sherbet
snack chips: potato, corn, etc.
snack crackers (high in fat)
soda pop, containing sugar
soft-serve ice cream
sorbet
sugar: white, brown, fructose (fruit sugar),
   maple, turbinado
sweet liqueurs and cordials (even if alcohol is
   permitted)
sweet pickles
sweet relish
sweet-and-sour sauces and glazes
sweetened, powdered drink mixes
sweet rolls (Danish pastry)
syrups
waffles
whipped cream, sugar-sweetened
whipped topping, nondairy, sugar-sweetened
wine coolers (contain sugar)

Preparing Meals

Cooking Methods

Except as directed in the recipes, do not use any fat, oil, butter, margarine, shortening, or high fat ingredients in cooking. This means that frying, and deep fat frying, are out!

Meat, poultry, fish, and seafood may be broiled, baked, roasted, steamed, stewed, microwaved, crock-potted, pressure-cooked, boiled, or barbecued (no fat or sugary glazes added). Food may also be sautéed in a nonstick skillet, which has been sprayed with vegetable cooking spray.

You may cook vegetables, potatoes, or rice in bouillon, consommé, or fat-free broth for flavor—no butter needed!

Permitted Seasonings

Salt is permitted, unless you are on a sodium-restricted diet. If you are, follow your doctor's advice. He or she may suggest that you omit salt and use a salt substitute and such alternative ingredients as salt-free bouillon.

Experiment with seasonings to make your food interesting. You may also use any of the following:

lemon juice	lime juice
mustard	horseradish
herbs	spices
sugar substitutes	baking powder
baking soda	unsweetened cocoa powder
coffee	beverages (sugar free)
decaffeinated coffee	vinegar
plain gelatin	sugar-free powdered
sugar-free gelatin mixes	drink mixes

Provided you are under no additional diet restrictions, you may use the following condiments in the specified amounts:

catsup, barbecue sauce, or chili sauce	1 tablespoon
cereal beverage, like Postum	1 tablespoon
relish	1 tablespoon
soy sauce	2 tablespoons
steak sauce	2 tablespoons

Permitted Beverages

You may drink all of the following you want:

regular or decaffeinated coffee, black*

tea, herbed tea, iced tea (sugar-free)*

* See Chapter 2 for information on the effects of caffeine.

Note: You may wish to use the milk allowed with the diet in the beverages above.

water (club soda or mineral water may be substituted)

sugar-free soda*   SF Koolaid   SF Tang

Sugar-Free Milk Drinks: Be aware that some of the sugar-free products, like the hot cocoa drinks, do contain milk. If you drink them, subtract them from your daily milk allowance.

Alcoholic Beverages Please do not drink any alcoholic beverages for the first two weeks. Thereafter, you should limit yourself to just one drink a day.

Use the following amounts:

1 ounce 80-proof liquor
or
4 ounces dry wine
or
1 light beer

Alcoholic beverages simply add calories to your diet, nothing more. And this diet changes your body chemistry, so one drink will have the effect of two.

Caution: Wine coolers and cream liqueurs contain sugar, and some drinks contain added fat. Coolers and punches sweetened with sugar are off limits. So are sweet and creamy after-dinner drinks that contain cream as well as sugar. Beware sugar-mixed drinks like whiskey sours and margaritas, and piña coladas that contain both sugar and fat in the form of sweetened coconut cream.

Dealcoholized wines and beers are also permitted (limited to one a day).

* See Chapter 2 for information on the effects of caffeine.

5 Putting It All Together: Sample Menus

Whether you love to cook or hate it, never eat out or never eat at home, adore spicy food or can't abide it, this diet can be adapted to fit your likes and lifestyle. Here are some menu suggestions to start you thinking:

MENU I

Breakfast

¼ small cantaloupe
⅓ cup low-fat cottage cheese
4 pieces of melba toast (rye or whole wheat)
    Beverage of your choice

Lunch

3 ounces turkey breast
1 small pita bread (whole wheat)
1 tablespoon high-protein, low-fat mayonnaise
    Lettuce
    Carrot or celery sticks or cucumber slices
1 large peach
    Beverage of your choice

Dinner

6 ounces barbecued beef flank steak or round steak, cooked in one of the marinade sauces
    Broiled tomato
    Green beans and carrots in broth
    (Phase Two: ½ cup brown or white rice cooked in bouillon)
    Fresh spinach salad with mushrooms and bean sprouts

   Buttermilk dressing
   Beverage of your choice

Snack

¾ cup berries
¾ cup plain yogurt with sweetener, if desired

MENU II

Breakfast

½ cup banana
½ cup raisin bran or Fiber One
 4 ounces skim milk
 1 ounce sliced, broiled ham
   Beverage of your choice

Lunch

   Seafood Fried Rice (see page 129)
   Lettuce and tomato salad, light dressing of your choice
   A crisp, red apple
   Beverage of your choice

Dinner

   Eggplant Parmesan (see page 145)
   (Phase Two: 1 thin slice Italian bread)
   Very large tossed salad
   Vinaigrette Dressing (see page 143)
   Beverage of your choice (Phase Two: 4 ounces of dry
     wine, optional)

Snack

   Melon in season
 1 ounce Yogurt Cheese (see page 201)

MENU III

Breakfast
   4 ounces orange juice
   1 poached egg
   1 slice of dry toast (raisin or whole wheat)
   Beverage of your choice

Lunch
   Sandwich: 2 ounces lean ham
   1 ounce part-skim mozzarella cheese
   2 slices of very thin bread or diet bread (toasted)
   Lettuce, 2 tablespoons Light and Creamy Russian
      Dressing (see page 141) on sandwich
   Garnish with raw vegetables and pickles
   ½ cup fresh or canned sugar-free pineapple
   Beverage of your choice

Dinner
   1 cup homemade or canned chicken broth with slivered
      carrots and celery
   Spicy Sweet and Sour Meatballs (see page 153) served
      with steamed cabbage, shredded
   Pickled beets in vinaigrette dressing
   (Phase Two: 1 small hard roll)
   Beverage of your choice

Snack
   ¾ cup plain yogurt
   2 tablespoons granola

MENU IV

Breakfast
8 ounces V8 juice
1 scrambled egg (or ¼ cup Eggbeaters) made with 2 ta-
    blespoons skim milk, ¼ teaspoon dry mustard,
    cooked in a nonstick pan sprayed with cooking spray
1 slice rye toast (dry)
Beverage of your choice

Lunch
3 ounces roast beef on small pita bread with mustard and
    lettuce
Green pepper ring, radishes, and green onion
1 orange
8 ounces low-fat milk or buttermilk

Dinner
Baked Boston scrod (5 ounces cooked) brushed with
    lemon juice and light mayonnaise
Steamed zucchini
(Phase Two: ½ cup green peas)
Cucumber in buttermilk or vinaigrette dressing
No-Cook Chocolate Mousse (see page 205)
Beverage of your choice

Snack
½ cup fresh or thawed raspberries
2 ounces pot style low-fat cottage cheese (⅓ cup)
Optional: sugar substitute to taste

MENU V

Breakfast
½ grapefruit
¼ cup granola
¾ cup plain yogurt
1 ounce boiled ham, lean
   Beverage of your choice

Lunch
1 cup low-fat cottage cheese served on lettuce with cut-up
      vegetables (cucumber, radishes, green onions, carrots,
      and celery)
½ toasted bagel (dry)
1 sweet, ripe pear
   Beverage of your choice

Dinner
   Chicken and Peppers (see page 158)
   Summer squash
2 bread sticks
   Large, herbed tossed salad with low-fat dressing
   Beverage of your choice

Snack
1 crisp apple
1 ounce farmer's or yogurt cheese

MENU VI

Breakfast

½ cup grapefruit juice
½ toasted whole wheat English muffin (dry)
 1 soft-cooked egg
  Sugar-free hot chocolate

Lunch

 3 ounces very lean corned beef, open-faced with 1 slice
    rye bread
  Prepared mustard
  Large dill pickle
½ bottle no-alcohol beer (or beverage of your choice)
 2 fresh plums

Dinner

  Oven Shish Kebob (see page 155) with 6 ounces lean
    lamb
  (Phase Two: ½ cup cooked Ramaki noodles)
  Salad of 1 cup grated carrots, diet dressing on a bed of
    lettuce
  Summer Squash, Turkish Style (see page 184)
  Luscious Lime Parfait (see page 214)

Snack

 1 whole wheat cracker
 1 ounce smoked mozzarella (or any processed low-fat
    cheese made from skim milk)

MENU VII: SUNDAY

Brunch

⅛ of Quiche Lorraine (see page 127)

Fruit salad of ½ orange, ¼ banana, ½ cup pineapple, ¼ cup plain yogurt as dressing—low-calorie sweetener optional

Broiled tomato half sprinkled with Parmesan cheese and sweet basil

½ bagel, spread with a teaspoon of cottage cheese blended with chives

Cinnamon coffee or herb tea

Afternoon Cocktail Hour

4 flavored melba toast

1 ounce Yogurt Cheese (see page 201)

Celery stuffed with ⅓ cup cottage cheese with chives

(Phase Two: 4 ounces dry white wine, or 1 ounce vodka, gin, scotch, or other hard liquor with water, club soda, or diet soda)

Dinner

5 ounces lean ham steak, broiled or sautéed in a nonstick skillet

(Phase Two: ½ baked sweet potato)

Mixed vegetables cooked in bouillon (carrots, Brussels sprouts, and cauliflower, for example)

Salad of onion, tomato and vinaigrette dressing on a bed of lettuce

Beverage of your choice

Snack (Dessert)

1 slice of Fruited Cheesecake (see page 209)

"I Hate to Cook" Menus

MENU I

Breakfast   (can be packed for work)
  1 orange
  6 saltines or four slices of melba toast (whole wheat or
      rye)
  1 ounce diet cheese
    Coffee, tea, or beverage of your choice

Lunch   (can be bought or brought from home)
    Sandwich: 3 ounces turkey
  2 slices reduced-calorie bread
  2 teaspoons "light" mayonnaise (pickles, lettuce, toma-
      toes permitted)
  1 apple, unpared, cut in wedges
    Beverage of your choice

Dinner
    One quarter of a roasted chicken (remove skin)—can be
      bought on the way home from work at the neighbor-
      hood deli
    Very large tossed salad (diet dressing only)
    (Phase Two: 2 bread sticks, whole wheat or rye)
  ⅛ of a honeydew melon (or other unsweetened fruit of
      your choice)
    Beverage of your choice

Snack
  ¾ cup of plain low-fat yogurt (add a few drops of vanilla,
      some crushed fruit, and sweeten to taste with sugar
      substitute if you like)

or

  1 single-serve packed sugar-free milk shake, prepared ac-
      cording to package directions

MENU II

Breakfast   (may be packed or eaten at home)
  4 ounces orange juice
  1 hard- or soft-cooked egg (or ¼ cup no-cholesterol sub-
    stitute, scrambled in a nonstick pan)
  1 slice raisin or whole wheat bread (plain or toasted)
    Beverage of your choice

Lunch   (can be bought or brought from home)
  1 cup vegetable soup
  1 plain hamburger with lettuce, tomato, pickle, etc., on ½
    bun or tucked in a 1-ounce pita pocket
  1 pear (may be brought from home)
    Beverage of your choice

Dinner
    Broiled, small (half-pound) raw boneless sirloin steak—
      equals 6 ounces cooked
    (Phase Two: small baked potato, topped with yogurt and
      chopped parsley, or chives)
  1 cup green beans, cooked (fresh, frozen, or canned)
    Salad (may be made fresh or left over from another
      meal)
    Beverage of your choice
    (Phase Two: 4 ounces dry red wine, optional)

Snack
    Skim milk
    Apple
  1 ounce cheese

MENU III

Breakfast
½ banana or ½ cup berries
½ cup Fiber One or ¾ cup Sun Flakes or 1 cup Special K
½ cup skim milk
   Beverage of your choice

Lunch   (bought or brought from home)
 3 ounces sliced lean ham and Swiss style diet cheese on 1
   slice of rye bread, with mustard
   Salad bar—2 tablespoons diet dressing
½ cup unsweetened fresh or canned fruit (no syrup)
   Beverage of your choice

Dinner
   Large salad Niçoise, including fresh vegetable, salad
      greens, raw green beans plus small 3-ounce can
      water-packed tuna
 2 hard-cooked eggs
 2 tablespoons low-calorie salad dressing
   (Phase Two: 4 pieces rye melba toast or crisp bread
      broken into croutons)
   Beverage of your choice
   (Phase Two: 8 ounces light beer, optional)

Snack
 1 crisp apple
 1 ounce Cheddar-style diet cheese
   Sugar-free hot cocoa, single-serving packet

MENU IV

Breakfast
½ grapefruit
1 ounce ham
1 slice bread (or ½ whole wheat bagel)
   Beverage of your choice

Lunch
   3 ounces corned beef (lean, round only) on 1 slice rye
      bread or 2 slices diet bread
   Pickle (sour or dill)
   Small salad
   (You can save your fruit for an afternoon break)
   Beverage of your choice

Dinner
   (Phase Two: 1 cup chicken noodle soup)
   6 ounces lean roast beef (bought at deli)
10-ounce package frozen broccoli, cooked and seasoned
      with lemon pepper
   Sliced tomato and cucumber salad
   Beverage of your choice

Snack
¾ cup plain yogurt
¼ cup fresh or frozen blueberries
   2 tablespoons granola
Optional: sugar substitute to taste

6 Carbohydrates, Protein, Fat, and Fiber: A Crash Course in Nutrition

You are what you eat—it's not just a saying. Food literally becomes you. Food is our primary tool for building strong bodies. Some knowledge of the basic facts of nutrition is helpful to everyone.

Except for the water we drink and the oxygen we breathe, the needs of the body can only be met by food. To nourish the body, food has three vital jobs:

- Provide fuel (calories) the body can burn to set free the energy needed for activity.
- Provide the building materials needed to make or maintain body tissue.
- Provide substances that help regulate body processes.

All foods are compounds, mixtures of chemicals found in nature, and these nourishing natural chemicals are known as nutrients. There are six classes of nutrients the body needs:

1. Carbohydrates
2. Proteins
3. Fats
4. Vitamins
5. Minerals
6. Water

All six are equally important.

Regardless of where you live on this earth—Kalamazoo, Katmandu, or Kuala Lumpur—no matter what the cuisine, you need all six nutrients.

The first three—carbohydrates, proteins, and fats—are the fuel nutrients, sources of calories. They are the only substances that the body can burn to supply energy for work and heat.

Let's deal with them one by one.

Carbohydrates

Carbohydrates are either simple sugars or more complex compounds, such as starch. All food carbohydrates except lactose (milk sugar) are formed in the vegetable kingdom.

The sweet taste of corn and peas is due to its natural sugar—sugar that will turn to starch when overripe. Sometimes it works the other way around. Some fruits, bananas for example, contain starch that turns to sugar on ripening. Carrots, beets, onions, winter squash, turnips, and sweet potatoes are all vegetables that contain appreciable amounts of natural sugar. Fruits are rich in natural sugar; that's why they're naturally sweet.

However, few foods in nature are as intensely sweet as refined white table sugar, or the candies, sweets, and snacks we have come to indulge in. In nature, sugar exists as part of a balanced "package." A sun-ripened peach plucked from the tree contains not only sugar but fiber, flavor, juice, and vitamins, particularly vitamin A. The natural sugar in fruits and vegetables comes copackaged with so much water and bulky fiber that it's difficult to overindulge in sugar from totally natural sources.

In refining sugar for table use, what we have done, essentially, is to separate the pure refined carbohydrate—the calories—from everything else of value in terms of nourishment and appetite control. The moisture, vitamin, and bulk are discarded. What remains is a refined white granulated substance with no nutritional value except calories. Refined sugar is simple carbohydrate, rapidly absorbed by the body.

What we tend to do with this refined white substance is to sprinkle and stir it into foods, making them sweeter than nature ever intended, thereby overburdening our bodies with an unnatural sugar load. This can have dire consequences for some people, contributing to the excessive rise in blood fats and blood sugar levels associated with heart disease and diabetes.

Sucrose and Fructose

Our sugar supply for table use and cooking comes chiefly from juices of the sugar cane or sugar beet. Sugar obtained from cane, sugar beets, and sap from the sugar maple tree are all sucrose, ordinary white table sugar. We often hear about another, supposedly healthier form of sugar: fructose, also known as fruit sugar. Granulated fructose and fructose syrups are sold in health food stores. High fructose corn syrup (refined from corn, as its name suggests) is being used in the food industry as a less expensive alternative to sucrose. The molecular differences between sucrose and fructose permit the latter to perform somewhat differently and give it a minor edge over sucrose as a sweetener for the weight conscious. Although both have identical calorie counts (16 per level teaspoon), fructose has more sweetening power than sugar when used with fruit or other acid-containing ingredients. Therefore you may need only half as much—half the calories' worth—of fructose to sweeten strawberry yogurt. However there would be no calorie savings in using fructose in vanilla mousse or chocolate cake; neither are acidic. Fructose is also absorbed more slowly than sucrose, making it less likely to raise blood sugar levels.

However fructose, like sucrose, is a refined carbohydrate. Like sucrose, it's pure calories. In this diet, where carbohydrates are kept in careful balance with protein in order to remedy water retention, there are no calories to waste on either fructose or sucrose. Only the natural fruit sugar that comes as part of a balanced package—an apple or orange, for example—is permitted. (Sugar substitutes are virtually free of calories and carbohydrates and may be used to augment sweetness for those with an unreformable sweet tooth!)

Honey, molasses, brown sugar, turbinado sugar

These are simply other forms of sugar, and are used by the body as sugar. They are also off limits on the 35-Plus Diet.

Starches

Starch is more complex than sugar. Starches are formed in plants by the union of many molecules of glucose, a form of sugar. Starch is the carbohydrate found in seeds, tubers, and roots where plants store it for future energy needs. In the plant, starch is laid down in granules coated with a celluloselike substance, and different plants have granules of characteristic size and shape.

When you cook starch granules, the cells absorb water, swell, and rupture. They are more easily digested in this state. Therefore, before starch can be used as a source of energy, it must be broken down into simple sugar. Cooking helps start the process so our bodies can finish the work. Our chief sources of starch are grains and the products made from them (breads, cereals, pastas, etc.) legumes (beans and peas), and certain tuber and root vegetables (potatoes and sweet potatoes).

Protein

Proteins are present in all living tissues—plant or animal—and they are essential to life. Proteins are a vital part of the nucleus and protoplasm of every cell. The human body is made up of a variety of specialized proteins, keratin, for example. The outer layers of skin, the hair, and the nails consist almost entirely of keratin.

The most native and abundant tissues of the body—the

muscles and glandular organs—are high in protein content. Blood, of course, carries the important protein hemoglobin in its red cells and several proteins in solution in fluid (plasma) portions.

Protein molecules are a kind of "mosaic" made up of nitrogen-containing compounds called amino acids.

Certain amino acids are said to be essential—that is, they must be already formed and present in the food. In reality, all amino acids are essential to the human body. However, the body can make at least some of them itself if necessary. For that reason, an amino acid is referred to as "essential" (indispensable) only if your body can't make it for itself.

It should be made clear that a vegetarian diet can provide adequate protein if a wide enough variety of vegetable proteins are eaten. In combination these can supplement each other to furnish adequate amounts of all essential amino acids.

It is extremely important to remember that protein, a valuable substance for both plants and animals, is not stored in large amounts. The supply should be *replenished daily*.

Fat

The high calorie count of fat (weight for weight more than twice that of carbohydrate or protein) means that relatively small amounts of fatty foods can quickly raise the caloric bottom line of the day's food intake. For that reason, fats are useful in a weight-*gaining* diet, or when it's desirable to have a high calorie intake with little bulk. Whenever you eat more calories than you burn off—whether the food is fat, protein, or carbohydrate—the extra calories are converted into body fat and stored in various parts of the body.

Fat deposits in the human body are good or bad according to whether they are moderate or excessive. Some fat under the skin and about the organs serves a useful purpose, historically as a reserve store of fuel in time of need. Moderate fat also help support organs, protect them from injury, and prevent loss of body heat. But an overfed person goes on storing fat that will never be needed.

Fiber

Fiber is not a true nutrient because much of it is indigestible, and therefore it doesn't "nourish." But vegetable fiber or cellulose is very important for a variety of reasons. Adding fiber foods to the diet is one of the best ways to cut calories without hunger. Fiber fills you up—not out. But fiber is more than bran flakes.

Fiber is an entire family of substances from a wide variety of vegetable sources. Different kinds of fiber produce different results and offer different benefits. To eat well and lose weight safely as well as enjoyably, you'll want to add a variety of fiber foods to the menu every day.

Fiber comes from vegetables, fruits, and whole grains. In fact, fiber is found *only* in "growing foods"—food from the earth—never in such animal foods as meat, fish, poultry, eggs, cheese, or milk. Cheap meat may be tough, stringy, and fibrous, but no animal food contains any dietary fiber whatsoever. That's because dietary fiber comes from the cell walls of plants. It includes such substances as cellulose, lignin, pectins, and gums.

Bran

Bran, the best known source of fiber, contains cellulose and lignin. But even bran offers a choice of sources. More than likely, the bran in your breakfast cereal or bran muffin comes from wheat, milled from the coarse outer layer of the wheat kernel. This is the dark, coarse part that's ground off in the manufacture of white bread flour. But bran can also be made from other grains: the outer layer of corn kernels, oats, soybeans, peas, or rice. Corn bran has a mild flavor and light color; rice bran is high in protein.

Whatever their source, all kinds of bran share a traditional claim to fame: the promotion of regularity. Constipation is the unpleasant and all-too-common outcome of a junk-food diet. Calorie-dense refined foods tend to compress and compact in the bowels. The addition of bran to the diet helps alleviate this uncomfortable condition by adding bulk or "roughage." Bulks helps to increase the speed of elimination.

You are also getting the benefits of bran when you eat whole grains, because the unprocessed grains have the valuable bran layer left intact.

Pectin

Other kinds of fiber come from fruits and vegetables. These are the water-retaining gums and pectins that are a normal part of the outer structure of plant cells. Pectin is best known for its ability to cause fruit purees to jell. Canners make use of this characteristic in the making of jelly. Just as pectin performs its action by holding water in suspension, gums and pectins do the same thing in the intestine, helping to forestall constipation and the production of hard dry compacted stools. Pectin is a natural softener. It's particularly abundant in the peels of apples and the skins of citrus fruits.

Health Benefits of a High-Fiber Diet

In recent years these beneficial regularity-promoting features of fiber have been shown to have other equally important health benefits. Because fiber helps to speed waste through human plumbing, internal body tissues spend less time in contact with potentially hazardous cancer-causing agents that may be in the food supply. And the gums and pectins found in fruits and vegetables help to prevent the absorption of cholesterol from animal foods, reducing blood cholesterol levels.

There are particular benefits for diabetics and hypoglycemia sufferers. Roughage helps to dilute and slow down the absorption of sugar into the bloodstream, thereby making it possible for some to reduce their insulin dependency. This same blood sugar regulating effect is important to dieters because blood sugar and insulin levels have an impact on hunger and sugar-cravings.

High-fiber dining is also said to help to lower cholesterol, lessen the risk of bowel cancer, and protect against colitis, appendicitis, hemorrhoids, and varicose veins.

A low-fat, high-fiber diet is recommended by the American Cancer Society, the American Heart Association, and the American Diabetes Association.

For 35-Plus Dieters, tricked by their metabolism into hungering for more food than they can utilize, the appetite-appeasement feature of fiber foods make them real winners. High-fiber foods are generally low-fat and calorie-light, puffed-up by nature with a healthy proportion of indigestible bulk. This bonus bulk satisfies the need to chew and fills the stomach, but it leaves the body without being metabolized or stored as unwanted body fat.

Enjoying fiber-rich dishes can help cut calorie intake and absorption. The fiber in food attracts and holds water, creating a sensation of fullness. Better yet, fiber speeds food through your system, helping to eliminate some of the nutrients before they can be completely absorbed.

The 35-Plus Diet is a low-fat, high fiber diet. When talking to my patients, I describe myself as a vegetable-pusher. I insist they eat more cooked as well as raw vegetables. Vegetables raise fiber intake and help fight the "hungries."

7 Calcium: A Woman's Special Problem

It's been drummed into us since childhood that milk and other calcium-containing foods are important to build strong bones and teeth during the growth period of youth. Now there's new understanding that an adequate intake of calcium is just as important in the adult years, to aid in the prevention of osteoporosis. This potentially crippling breakdown of bone tissue in midlife and beyond is truly a women's disease. The fact that it does attack chiefly women—middle aged and older women at that—may explain why osteoporosis never garnered as much attention, until recently, as male-threatening heart disease.

It's quite common for women approaching midlife to begin suffering from a slow but relentless washing away of bone. This is the primary cause of such bone deformities as the dowager's hump in elderly women and also makes the bones more likely to break with injury. While the causes of this bone loss are still not completely understood, several important factors have been identified:

1. Lack of exercise. Without sufficient exercise to put stress on the bones, they will soften regardless of what else is done. The exercise must be weight-bearing. That's why walking has outranked swimming as the ideal, all-purpose exercise.
2. Lack of calcium in the diet. For various reasons, mature women often do not take in enough calcium to allow the body to keep the bones strong.
3. Lack of female hormone (estrogen). After menopause,

women become much more prone to osteoporosis. There is evidence that estrogen replacement can help reverse this. However, taking estrogen may increase the risk of cancer of the uterus. Consequently, putting a postmenopausal woman on estrogens is not an automatic treatment but is done only after the woman and her physician carefully evaluate the risks and benefits of the individual case.

4. Other factors such as race and heredity. The risk of osteoporosis is highest in white women and lowest in black men.

Exercising Care for Your Bones

We can't change our race and sex. And we'll want to think long and hard about taking hormones. But we can begin right now taking steps—literally and figuratively—to preserve our bones. Even if you are a total couch potato, you can begin today by taking a walk to the end of the block. Tomorrow add another block. And continue adding blocks until you are taking a one-hour walk every day. After that you can begin working on your speed, gradually increasing the number of blocks you can walk in one hour. This simple fitness program is easy to maintain anywhere, no matter where you live, work, or travel. If need be, you can even walk around the same block several times, in circles, or up and down the same block. Walking indoors for an hour has the same effect; if necessary, in bad weather you might walk the corridors of your office building. I know a frequent flyer who walks airline terminals between flights.

Fighting osteoporosis should be reason enough to begin an exercise program. When you add it to all the other, perhaps better-known motivations, it's apparent that exercise is of paramount importance to the 35-Plus Woman. Consider these other benefits:

- You'll help protect your heart. As women approach mid-life, they need to remember that the heart-saving hormonal advantage they have had over men will eventually decline. Past menopause, women's risk of heart disease is similar to that experienced by men.
- You'll feel better. Exercise is a great mood elevator. It's easier to remain on a diet when your outlook is optimistic.
- You'll be less hungry. Inactivity impairs the body's natural appetite control mechanism.
- You'll lose weight faster if you exercise.
- You'll look thinner at the same weight than if you didn't exercise.
- You'll speed up your metabolism, lessening the likelihood that you'll regain the weight lost.

Adding Calcium to Your Diet

To maintain good bone strength, you need 1,000 to 1,500 mg of calcium a day in your diet. The best source of calcium is dairy products.

Dairy Products	Calcium
8 ounces skim milk	359 mg
8 ounces whole milk	298 mg
1 ounce hard cheese	218 mg
1 ounce slim soft cheese	158 mg
½ cup cottage cheese (low fat)	105 mg
1 cup yogurt (skim milk plain)	293 mg

Nondairy Products	Calcium
½ cup green leafy vegetables (broccoli, kale, collards, turnip greens, mustard greens, dandelion greens)	50–180 mg
1 cup whole wheat flour	49 mg
1 cup white enriched flour	20 mg
½ cup dried beans	75–150 mg

Ideally, a well-planned diet should provide enough calcium to meet minimum daily requirements; however, experience has shown that with older people, many of whom have trouble digesting milk and some milk products, it may be difficult to take in adequate calcium through meals alone. If you are unable to get 1,000 to 1,500 mg calcium a day in your diet, you should seriously consider using a calcium supplement.

Of the many calcium supplements available, calcium carbonate is inexpensive and effective. An excellent and inexpensive source of calcium carbonate is Tums. Four regular strength or three extra strength Tums should provide all the extra calcium you need, but if it fails to work for you—some women experience an uncomfortable gassy feeling—experiment with other preparations. If you are going to use a calcium supplement please note the following:

1. Avoid high-priced products, particularly those sold in health food stores. They are no more safe or effective than plain calcium carbonate.
2. Anyone with a history of kidney stones should check first with her physician before taking extra calcium.

On the other hand, if you cannot tolerate supplements, then you should manipulate the protein allowance in the diet to increase your calcium intake. Use three servings (3 ounces) of your daily protein allowance in the form of low-fat cheese. When the cheese is added to the 1 cup of milk called for by the 35-Plus Diet, that will give you 4 servings of milk foods a day.

Vitamin D

Vitamin D is required by the body, in addition to calcium, for the formation of strong bones. Vitamin D is found in the diet in dairy products. It is also found in large amounts in fish oils. Your body can manufacture its own Vitamin D if you are exposed to enough sunlight.

If you cannot tolerate dairy products and are not exposed to much sunlight, you may obtain extra Vitamin D by taking *one* multiple vitamin tablet a day. This should be taken with a meal. If taken in excessive amounts, Vitamin D can be *toxic* so do not exceed recommended dosage.

Substances That Interfere With Body Calcium Levels

Certain substances tend to reduce body calcium levels by acting in a variety of ways. Those substances include

antacids that contain aluminum, such as Maalox, Mylanta, Gelusil, Amphojel

cortisone type drugs in large doses

caffeine in large amounts (coffee, tea, cola beverages, some pain relievers)

nicotine (tobacco)

alcoholic beverages

fad diets very high in protein

None of these substances will cause harm with occasional use. However, heavy users should discuss their calcium needs with their physicians.

8 The Pleasure Principle

There's an aspect of the 35-Plus Woman's life that I suspect may have subtle but profound effects on her physical well-being as well as her emotions. I call it the pleasure principle. There are no scientific studies to support my guess, but my observations tend to suggest that the less of it a woman has in her life—pleasure, that is—the more likely she is to run into problems, including weight problems. Yes, I am talking about sexual fulfillment, but that's just one of a whole range of pleasures that I sense are sadly missing from some women's lives.

But let's talk about that one first.

I don't conduct research into the sex lives of my patients. In fact I never bring up the topic. But in the course of seeing hundreds of women in my office and in classes, I sometimes do get to know quite a bit about their private lives. What's clear to me is that many women, including many young women in their thirties, have simply ceased to function sexually.

Some women confide in distress that their husbands are no longer interested in them. Even more worrisome, perhaps, are the women who are themselves no longer interested.

Here's a tipoff to the sexually dead relationship. When I ask a woman how her husband feels about her weight, she replies, "He's used to me." As if she were wallpaper.

Sexual Disconnection

Why is it, do you suppose, that these women seem so turned off, so out of touch with their sexuality? And which came first? The weight problem followed by sexual disconnection. Or did they cease being sexual beings and then gain weight? This isn't a test; I honestly don't know the answer myself. But I find it worth considering.

It's possible to imagine a couple of different scenarios of how this sexual extinction might come to be.

In one scene, she puts on weight, and that turns him off. To avoid sexual confrontation, he falls asleep on the sofa or stays out late. Or hangs out at the office or the neighborhood bar. He may drink excessively or otherwise behave boorishly to make himself so unattractive that the sexual abstinence seems like her idea. Or he may simply rebuff her advances, something so humiliating to a woman that she quits asking—and ultimately quits wanting. To save her ego she becomes sexually numb.

Or in another variation of the same play, she puts on weight and turns herself off. She feels flabby and sexually unattractive. In the bedroom even with the lights off, she's so focused on her imagined physical shortcomings that she's completely unable to respond to her mate's advances. Sex becomes an ordeal for both of them, and they quit trying.

And then there's another intriguing and even more complex scenario: the one in which she—or he or they—lose interest in sex first. And then she gains weight. This is particularly fascinating for the number of questions it raises. Why do some people turn off sexuality in the prime of life? Is it particular to the relationship—they're not getting along for whatever reasons—or is it a widespread symptom of the fast-trackers' overextended appointment book? And why do some women respond to the stress in their lives and the absence of sexual fulfillment by gaining weight? Is it simply a matter of substituting chocolate bars for sexual pleasure? Or is it more complicated? Does the premature shutdown in sexuality induce—prematurely—at least some of the hormonal changes that contribute to weight gain?

I can't pretend to know the answers or even all the questions about how the pleasure principle relates to 35-Plus weight problems, but I do know that things tend to change dramatically in this regard as the excess weight is lost. It's truly a delight for me to observe one of these sexually asleep women beginning to stir and emerge from her hibernation. She starts wearing makeup again and styling her hair. The first outward manifestations may be something so simple as nail polish or wearing a dress to class instead of the same old baggy jeans or stretchpants. Quite simply she starts looking prettier and smiles more. She may let it be known, through jokes and innuendo, that she's sexually alive again.

If I had to give advice on this aspect, I'd go with the likely. I'd suggest that keeping one's sexuality alive—by whatever means—is probably beneficial in ways that we may not yet understand. The mind and body work in concert and the counsel to "use it or lose it" probably relates to sex as well as exercise.

The first step in fulfilling this prescription is often simply to make the time. I am honestly aghast at the burdens some 35-Plus Women are carrying and their grim determination to be superwoman.

Permissible Pleasures

Sexual fulfillment is only one of a whole range of pleasures that may be missing from some women's lives. With the responsibilities some of these women carry—attending to demanding mates, raising children, caring for parents, maintaining houses, competing in corporations or professions, building for the future—there seems to be no "self" time left over. No time to indulge the senses except in the kitchen or when they sit down to a meal. Music? For many, the only time to listen to music is in the elevator on the way to the office. Movies? Flowers? Art? Leisure time is curtailed for the executive, and the creative expressions that homemakers used to enjoy as part of their job description are left undone or assigned to professionals.

Food

For many of these overweight women, even food is not to be enjoyed. Those who overeat the most often enjoy it the least.

The whole language of food in the diet world is one of enmity, of mortal combat between good and evil, virtue and temptation, bean sprouts and butter cookies. In the rhetoric of dieting, snacks and sweets abound everywhere, waiting in ambush, calorically armed with fattening ingredients, always ready for a sniper assault on the unwary weight watcher. For the person brainwashed by the media into thinking that excess weight is a burden of shame, the simple act of *enjoying* food is taken away. That's why fat people prefer not to eat with other people and generally feign disinterest in food—when anyone's watching. Underfed in public so that hunger is unsatisfied, the guilty fat person waits until nobody's looking to have her way with food, furtively and with a sense of shame and guilt. And the punitive remorse that follows such secret binges is especially damaging—the self flagellation, the inner dialogues: "You're a worthless glutton. You deserve to be fat!" It's certain that our mental and emotional attitudes affect the chemistry of our bodies: who knows what effect such attitudes have on our metabolism? Most of the small and elite group of winning losers—people who do take weight off and keep it off for good—have succeeded in making food one of many pleasures—not an enemy. Their winning approach is characterized by a positive embrace of healthy nonfattening foods rather than a negative rejection of forbidden foods. Since both sets of people work with the same

two lists, OK and Not OK, at first glance the differences
may not seem so readily apparent.

But there are crucial differences in the point of view here.
On the one hand there's an upbeat aggressive assertion of
one's right to the enjoyment of eating, a celebration of
wholesome foods. Contrasted with that is the defensive
self-punishing posture of the person who is perennially
fending off food, who never gives herself permission to
enjoy what she eats.

Please Yourself

The point to be made here is that pleasing oneself—in
many ways, and on many levels—is important. The 35-Plus
Woman with a weight problem should take the time to get
her full measure of pleasure in as many nonfattening ways
as possible, not only at home but wherever life takes her.
Making the time for small pleasures—concert listening,
gallery hopping, antique shopping, floating on a rubber raft
reading a trashy novel—it's your right.

And if some task must remain untended so you can make
a little time for youself, so what?

9 Questions and Answers About the 35-Plus Diet

Q. How much weight should I lose?

A. Enough to bring yourself down to a healthy and attractive size—whatever suits your age, your life-style, and the way you want to feel and look. But set reasonable goals for yourself. Not everyone can look like Cher—or should want to.

From the onset of puberty, a woman's shape is sculpted from fat as well as muscle. Women have a different body composition from men because women are built for childbearing. Our whole physiology is geared toward providing—storing—nourishment. In other words, being "fat" compared with today's role models.

A mature woman is courting disappointment and distress if she sets her sights on achieving the boyish body contours of the sixteen-year-old models pictured in *Vogue*. You must remember that many of these girls were *born* skinny—that's one reason why they became models. And very few women entering midlife can maintain the kinds of bodies you see on *Dynasty*. If you are a glamorous actress, it is in your best interest, financial and otherwise, to expend the enormous effort it undoubtedly takes—the time and money, the extreme self-denial, even the plastic surgery—to maintain these bodies.

If you are not naturally thin, not a professional entertainer, consider carefully the costs to your health and happiness of trying to maintain a silhouette that previous generations would have regarded as emaciated. Lose enough weight to be your own best self.

Q. What should I weigh?

A. This is a question every patient asks. They're usually pretty shocked by my refusal to drag out the height-weight tables. I explain that this is truly an individual matter.

Not all women who are 5 feet 2 inches—or 5 feet 4 inches or 5 feet 8 inches—are going to look alike or weigh alike. Only identical twins have the same genetic makeup. And it's your genes that dictate what kind of shape you will have—just as surely as they decided your eyes would be blue.

The only one who can determine your "correct" weight —the weight at which you look, feel, and function best—is *you.* In fact, you probably have a pretty good idea about what that weight is right now. That's the weight that should be your "goal," not a number decided by a chart or diet counselor!

Actually, the Metropolitan Life Insurance weight tables have recently become more liberal, with wider revised ranges. Nevertheless, some diet groups are enslaved by rigid height-weight charts, even to the point of requiring that their members get a written excuse from their doctors to stop dieting at 135 if their chart says 120. At Kaiser Permanente the doctors send these patients to me for evaluation before signing the "permission" letter.

When I question these women before I write the letter, I ask them what was the last time they weighed 120. They usually tell me that it was in junior or senior high!

It is simply a mistake to imagine that your "correct" weight is what the scales registered twenty or more years ago when you were an adolescent. Your own feelings, your own ability to function are much surer guides than a height-weight table.

Q. What about sudden weight gain?

A. Sometimes a woman puts on a great deal of weight in a short time. A change in life-style may be the cause: A busy homemaker, used to running after active children, may gain weight when she takes a job sitting at a desk all day. Or a woman with an active job may put on weight quickly when she finds herself suddenly retired. Others gain when they stop smoking or when an injury curtails an active sports life. In these circumstances it's distressingly easy to put on ten to thirty pounds in a very short period. These are the pounds we go after in short order to take off as soon as we can. The 35-Plus Diet does a very good job of this.

Q. I plan to keep on dieting until I lose an extra 10 pounds as a safety margin. Do you think that's a good idea?
A. No, it's not. It's counterproductive—more likely to lead to weight gain than remaining a few pounds *above* your goal weight. Here's why:

People sometimes diet themselves to superskinniness because they think it will give them leeway to eat whatever they want when they go "off" the diet. If you go back to eating the way you used to eat, you'll go back to what you used to weigh. Guaranteed!

In fact, if you've been thirty pounds or more overweight for a number of years, it's better to be a few pounds above your "ideal" weight, because you know you can never go off your maintenance diet.

To maintain your weight loss, use Phase Three. This phase, you'll note, is similar to Phase Two of the diet, with two to three servings of fat added to each day's menu. Phase Three also gives you the weekend off (or any two days you choose) to depart from the discipline of the diet, within reason, by indulging in foods not permitted on the diet days.

But remember that the purpose of dieting is to replace bad eating habits with new, healthier ones.

Q. Does the 35-Plus Diet ever not work?
A. Occasionally I will come upon a patient who is not los-

ing weight. When I question her in detail, I discover that she has been trying to lose weight faster by not eating all the food on the 35-Plus Diet. She'll tip me off by complaining that the less she eats the less she loses. And, of course, she's right!

Almost invariably I discover that the patient has unwittingly changed the ratio of food groups we set up. As a result she was eating less protein than was prescribed, and therefore more carbohydrate in relationship to protein. True, she was eating fewer calories. but as one of our subjects demonstrated on the control diet, it was possible to *gain* 1¼ pounds with a daily intake of only 950 calories! Despite a balanced low-calorie diet, she ended up weighing more than she did when she started.

Hidden fats can also wreak havoc with the diet. On top of our national fondness for sugar, we Americans also take a great deal of excessive calories in the form of fat. Remember, fat has twice as many calories weight for weight as carbohydrates or proteins. We take most of these fats as hidden calories—in fast foods, pastries, sauces, condiments, salad dressings, and the like. Since fat occurs naturally in many nutritious foods—especially meats and dairy products—extras and toppings can quickly add percentage points (and calories) to the 35-Plus Diet equation.

Q. What about the extra-petite person under five feet?
A. If you are a person smaller in stature, you *may* need to cut calories to 700–800 a day by reducing serving sizes 10 to 20 percent. It's essential, however, that you keep to the prescribed ratio of carbohydrates-proteins-fats and not simply cut out or reduce one group or another.

Q. Is this a good diet for everyone?
A. I don't recommend the diet for pregnant women, nursing mothers, or anyone who is recuperating from a debilitating disease.

A woman who was at one of my classes wanted to know if her daughter could use the diet. The daughter was 2½ months pregnant, and her mother felt this diet was better balanced than what the young woman normally ate. It may well have been. Nevertheless I suggested she come to see me for a prenatal diet instead.

Q. What about diabetics?

A. If you are an adult-onset/diabetic and not insulin-dependent, you may use the diet if you check with your doctor. I do use it in my practice, but only with the approval of the patient's physician.

Q. I'm trying to reduce my sodium intake. Could I use this diet?

A. That depends. The basic 35-Plus Diet aims to achieve diuresis (flushing out excess fluid) *without* sodium restriction. If you've been put on a sodium-restricted regimen by your doctor for medical reasons, you should get his or her advice before you make any changes. But if your doctor approves, or if you merely wish to cut salt intake for nonmedical reasons, you can use the diet and simply eliminate salt or salty ingredients from the recipes.

Q. What about the children? Will it harm them to eat my diet dinners?

A. Main courses made with lean protein foods, fresh vegetables, whole grains and fruit are healthy choices for everyone, so there's no reason why your youngsters can't share your meals—with some modifications. *Growing children need more calories than you do,* and this need should be met with extra servings of bread, pasta, milk, fruit and unsaturated fats.

I see a great many pitiable youngsters who are already morbidly obese in their early teens. Most of them come from homes where the family diet is high in fat and refined

sugar. If your child appears to be developing a weight problem, you should not delay seeking medical attention.
*Weight loss for children and adolescents should be under
medical supervision.*

*Q. Doesn't it take time to diet? I'm too busy to prepare spe-
cial recipes.*

A. Let me tell you about one of my success stories. A strik-
ingly attractive and very successful young woman in her
thirties, a CPA with her own busy firm, came to my program after the holidays. She could no longer fit into her
Brooks Brothers suits, but tax time was approaching, and
she was worried about how she'd find time for her diet.

I showed her how she could do this diet with little or no
cooking and also accommodate her travel needs. She called
me late in April after taxes to say, "Let me make your day,
Mrs. Spodnik. I've lost thirty pounds, and I feel and look
wonderful." She related she was ready for Phase Three.
Phase Three also accommodates itself to busy people's
lives.

*Q. What's the difference between premenstrual and premen-
opausal water retention?*

A. To put it briefly: One goes away by itself, the other does
not. The cyclical ebbing and flowing of hormones in
younger women can cause premenstrual syndrome. The
symptoms may include cramps, headache, depression, and
food cravings, especially sugar cravings that cause temporary fluid retention and water weight gain before the onset
of the monthly period. When the period begins, the symptoms abate, only to recur the following month. After thirty-
five, however, the *general* level of female hormones begins
to drop, body composition changes, insulin levels increase,
and the body retains more fluid. But this type of water
retention, unlike the premenstrual bloating, doesn't depart
at the end of the month.

Q. Why do I have so much trouble trimming my waist?

A. The thickening waistlines that some healthy active attractive women develop in their forties—despite regular exercise programs—is definitely peculiar to the 35-Plus hormone syndrome. Because these women are active and fit, with generally good muscle tone, the weight literally "settles" in the one place left where fat can accumulate. They tend to put on eight or ten pounds in the waist area, like a little paunch, and they can't lose it. Whatever they used to do doesn't work anymore. They're into fitness, looking good and feeling good. They do everything they've been told they're supposed to do—nutritionally and exercise-wise—including pasta salads instead of meat. But they have no waistline. They may even say, "I weigh the same, but everything has slipped: I used to have a twenty-six inch waist and now it's twenty-eight or thirty. And I haven't gained an ounce. But none of my belts fit anymore!" This is all dictated by hormones. While it's true that dieting can't "spot-reduce," this particular problem is one area where diet rather than exercise is the answer.

Q. What about high blood pressure—hypertension?

A. I have patients who have been faithful followers of the 35-Plus Diet for the past several years and with successful weight loss have been able to get off medication for hypertension. I must stress that this was under their doctors' care, not on their own. If you have high blood pressure, be sure to discuss weight control with your physician and follow his or her advice.

Q. My cholesterol is high, too. Can this diet help me with that?

A. Anyone with a weight problem should have both cholesterol and triglyceride levels checked and follow her doctor's counsel about bringing blood fat levels down to a healthy reading. Discuss weight control and this diet with your phy-

sician. In my practice, I have found that the 35-Plus Diet
succeeds in reducing cholesterol levels as well as weight for
many of my patients. But your doctor should be the one to
advise in your particular case.

Q. Is it ok to eat any kind of seafood?
A. From a weight-loss perspective, yes. Virtually all fish
and seafood are relatively low in fat and calories. Even the
so-called "fat" fishes like mackerel and bluefish are calorie-light compared with some popular cuts of meat.
Moreoever, the latest word from the nutrition researchers
is that the natural oil in some fish may even help lower
cholesterol. But if your physician has advised against fish
for any reason, then naturally you should follow his instruc-
tions.

Q. What about the cholesterol in shellfish?
A. For years some shellfish was believed to be high in cholesterol, and people were told not to eat very much of it,
particularly if they had high cholesterol levels. Now all
that's changed. The latest word from the American Heart
Association is that you should eat all kinds of seafood, but
limit the use of shrimp, lobster, or sardines to no more than
one serving per week. Clams, oysters, mussels, scallops,
and crab are now permissible, no longer on their limited
list. Like fish, most shellfish is extremely low in fat and
calories.

Q. Do you advise taking estrogen?
A. I do not advise for or against taking estrogen—this is a
decision to be made by you and your physician.

*Q. Do you recommend bonemeal or dolomite as calcium
supplements?*
A. No. In fact, in my classes I usually warn people against
bonemeal and dolomite; it's my understanding that they
may be contaminated with lead.

Q. When should I take the vitamins you recommend?

A. Take your multivitamin/minerals with the largest meal of the day—vitamins and minerals are best absorbed in the presence of other nutrients. If you are taking Tums as a form of calcium carbonate, I do suggest splitting the four per day and taking two shortly after one meal and the other two with another meal.

Q. How does the 35-Plus Diet work over the long term?

A. Very well, if you stick to it. Keeping excess weight off permanently is the real goal of every dieter. Unfortunately, as you probably know from your own experience, virtually all diets fail. If you have lost weight and regained it, you're in the company of the majority of dieters. The failure statistics are truly depressing: Only one person in twenty manages to lose weight—and keep it off for five years or more!

In my thirty years as a dietician, I've had ample opportunity to observe those statistics with many kinds of diets. They may take weight off, but they don't solve the underlying problems or aid the dieter in keeping weight off. Until this diet. This diet *works* for the 35-Plus Woman. And it equips her with the means for keeping weight off, for good.

In the first place, Phase Three solves the discouraging water-weight rebound that inevitably follows in other diet programs. The sudden weight regain that generally results after going "off" a diet is demoralizing and dispiriting. At this point, many people abandon weight control and efforts altogether and binge their way back to their original weight —plus a few pounds more.

Phase Three provides the successful weight loser with the tools for maintaining weight loss permanently while continuing with a normal and satisfying life that includes the enjoyment of food and food-related pleasures such as holidays, parties, travel, and dining out. She can enjoy restaurants, ethnic foods, and wine with dinner. Phase Three is flexible, easy to follow, and undemanding. A person who enjoys cooking and food exploration can fit her interests into Phase Three. On the other hand, a person who rarely cooks and eats out often isn't burdened with diet demands that require specially prepared meals at home. There's no need to count calories.

Equally important, in addition to weight control, Phase Three addresses other special nutritional needs and concerns of women approaching midlife. It is anticancer, antiosteoporosis, antidiabetic, antihypertension, and antiheart disease.

Q. I'm on the road nearly all the time. How can I possibly stay on a diet?

A. It is not too difficult to stay on the diet while traveling if you'll take a few precautions.

Many fine restaurants now offer special entrees for the dieter that are free of sauces, butter, or added oil. In most instances the menu will pretty accurately describe what's going to be on the plate, without a lot of seductive and mysterious descriptions of its garnish and preparation. Even fast-food restaurants are now offering salads and other alternatives to the 800-calorie double cheeseburger. Any restaurant worth its salt should be willing to prepare food to your order: substituting a green vegetable or salad for french fries or simply omitting the biscuits and gravy and other fattening side dishes that can be all too tempting when they're actually before you on the plate. Ask the waiter to *remove* the bread basket and butter if he brings them around. Don't be shy about making such requests. There are too many weight-conscious Americans out there, making similar demands, for you to feel you're out of place doing the same.

Juggle your daily carbohydrate allowances so that they can be included in the meal which will be the most difficult to plan or control. You'll want to have as many options open to you as possible.

If you're in the car a lot, take some fruit along or even pack a small insulated bag with carrot and celery sticks, diet soda, food for lunch. Small sealed plastic containers filled with a gel and kept in the freezer—sold at hardware and variety stores—will keep the food chilled and safe for hours without the mess of ice. Individual tins of water-packed tuna now come with pull-tops and you can purchase small containers of low-fat cottage cheese either plain or with bits of vegetable added. When you're buying and eating on the run, check the label both for ingredients and for size of the portion. If it's twice what you need and you'll be tempted to eat it all at one sitting, *throw out the extra before* you begin your meal. You're not "keeping good food from going to waste" by dumping it on yourself when your body doesn't need it, and eating it yourself is certainly not going to help the other hungry folk in the world. Forget the "clean plate club": you've resigned!

Airline food presents a more formidable problem. The fact that it's usually unappetizing may help you forgo the airline meal for a better meal later. Or you may be able to order a dietetic meal if you phone the airline in advance: it may not be exactly what you want but you should be spared the floury sauces and have a fair idea of what's on your plate. If the airline can't accommodate you, don't be afraid to bring along a meal from home. Try to make it a treat: vegetable nibbles, your favorite fruit, a good broiled steak chilled and sliced thin so you can roll the slices and eat them with your fingers, your favorite dill pickles. Your seatmate will be envious.

Breakfast at a restaurant is easy: you should be able to order almost anything that you would prepare at home. But beware of filled omelets and scrambled eggs, which the cook will probably prepare with butter.

When ordering dinner, avoid fried foods, sauces, and gravy. You could have lean roast beef, filet mignon, broiled fish, or roast chicken with the skin removed. You could

have, with the meat, half a large baked potato with a vegetable side dish and salad. Avoid rich salad dressings, sour
cream, butter, anything sweetened with sugar. Some fat
may be on the broiled fish or chicken. If possible, request
that it be broiled with a minimum of oil. For dessert, have
fresh fruit or save your allotted drink (have a Perrier or
Pellegrino with lime before dinner) and have brandy and
coffee instead of dessert. Avoid liqueurs, which are loaded
with sugar.

10 Twenty-five Ways to Make Your Diet Work Better

1. Don't skip meals. If you pass up breakfast, you'll only overeat at lunch—or snack midmorning on unhealthy foods. Make breakfast the time for filling, high-fiber fruit, whole-grain cereal, and calcium-rich skim milk.

2. Take a walk before or after dinner. It's the best exercise for using calories and controlling appetite—much better than sporadic strenuous workouts.

3. Always eat the most filling, least fattening foods first— salad before the meal, not after.

4. Never reward yourself with food. The food payoff habit makes you think you're hungry whenever life gives you a hard time.

5. Make time to eat properly—forget the grazing craze. Gobbling and snacking on the run only leave you hungry and unsatisfied.

6. Enjoy what you eat. *Focus* on your food. Savor the flavor of every morsel. Get a full measure of enjoyment from every bite.

7. Shop for food after meals, not before. If you go to the supermarket hungry, you'll be tempted to buy more than you need.

8. Make a careful shopping list. And don't buy any food not on it.

9. When you bring home raw vegetables from the grocery store, clean and prepare them immediately. Carrot and celery sticks, broccoli and cauliflower florets will keep

very well if stored, well-drained, in a big plastic bag in your refrigerator. Having these handy is a great time-saver and you'll be particularly grateful for them if you have a sudden snack attack.

10. Avoid sugar and sugar-containing foods or beverages. Sugar raises your insulin level and creates hunger.

11. Satisfy your sweet tooth with fresh fruit. The natural fruit sugar in fruit is handled differently by the body. And fresh fruit contains appetite-appeasing fiber and pectin that hold moisture and create stomach-filling bulk.

12. Learn to eat just once. One brownie instead of a whole batch. That's what maintenance is all about.

13. Fill up on liquids. Think you're hungry? Have a big glass of ice water or a hot bowl of soup before dinner.

14. Don't eat between meals. If three squares plus a snack means you find yourself tempted in between, schedule additional snacks made up of raw vegetables.

15. Make sure you eat your fill of the high-fiber foods your diet permits: whole grains, fresh fruits and vegetables, beans, bran, and other filling fare. They fill you up faster and help keep you feeling full longer.

16. Add foods with a high water content to your menu: lettuce, most salad vegetables, many fruits (especially melons), sugarless gelatin desserts.

17. Don't use food as a tranquilizer. Chewing to relieve tension is a habit that originates in infancy. If you can't beat the urge to chew, keep celery sticks handy.

18. Forget about it! Try not to think, talk, or read about food between meals. Avoid food ads and discussions of favorite recipes or restaurants.

19. Slow down. If you're the first one done eating, you'll be eyeing second helpings while others are finishing.

20. Avoid bland and boring foods; focus on the spicy, well-seasoned foods that make an impression on your taste buds.

21. Make your meals a habit: Eat in the same place at the same time as often as feasible.

22. Use your head! Use thought control techniques to "turn off" the attraction of fattening foods. If you visualize a jelly doughnut as glutted with artery-clogging fat and sugar, it will have less appeal.

23. Avoid "bad companions"—people and places that cause you to consume foods you shouldn't eat. If you can't walk by the bakery without the fragrance of cinnamon buns taking control of your brain, walk on the other side of the street.

24. If one scoop is never enough, don't bring quarts of ice cream into the house. When you're in maintenance and have a "vacation day" from the diet, have your ice cream at the soda fountain, and order a single scoop. Save such splurges for food you really love.

25. Keep food out of sight, wrapped in foil rather than see-through plastic.

II The 35-Plus Diet Cookbook

A Note on the Recipes

The number of people the recipe will serve is indicated at the beginning of each recipe. Also indicated are the number of "servings" or units from the various food groups—as defined in Chapter 3 and the 35-Plus Diet Food Lists in Chapter 4—that the recipe provides. These servings are calculated per portion (that is, per person served) at the end of each recipe, and the following abbreviations are used:

Fruit	*FR*
Grain/Starch	*ST*
Lean Protein	*PR*
Light Vegetables	*VEG*
Skim Milk/Yogurt	*ML*

11 Breakfast and Brunch Ideas

Many of the recipes in this breakfast and brunch section could also serve as lunch or supper dishes.

Two Simple Methods for Cooking Eggs Without Added Fat

Poached Eggs

Pour water into a saucepan to the height of 2 inches. The secret to poaching eggs successfully is to heat the water only to a simmer, *not* to a hard boil, which will break up the egg. Break each egg individually into a saucer. Tilt the saucer so that the egg slips into the water. Simmer egg 3 to 5 minutes, depending on size. Remove with a slotted spoon.

Each egg provides: 1 PR

Scrambled Eggs (or egg substitute)

Beat 1 tablespoon water or skim milk into each egg (¼ cup thawed liquid no-cholesterol egg substitute may be used in place of each egg). Spray a nonstick skillet with cooking spray; add no fat. Heat skillet over medium heat. When hot, add eggs. Use a wooden spoon or heat-proof rubber scraper to lift and move eggs gently as they cook. Continue stirring until the desired texture is reached. Remove from heat and season to taste.

Each egg (or equivalent egg substitute) provides: 1 PR

OMELET   Serves 1

2 eggs or ½ cup no-   2 tablespoons water
    cholesterol egg   Salt and pepper
    substitute

Fork-blend 2 eggs (or ½ cup no-cholesterol egg substitute) with 2 tablespoons water. Season to taste with salt and pepper, if desired. Spray a small nonstick omelet pan with cooking spray. Heat the pan over medium heat. When the pan is hot, add the egg mixture. Cook 30 seconds without disturbing, then shake the pan gently. Use a spatula or heat-proof rubber scraper to lift the eggs so that the uncooked portion can run beneath. When eggs are set, tilt the pan and lift one edge of the cooked omelet with the spatula or scraper. Gently roll the omelet over and out of the pan on to a warm plate.

Each portion (1 recipe) provides: 2 PR

One-pan Western Omelet   Serves 2

4 eggs or equivalent no-   3 tablespoons minced
    cholesterol egg   onion
    substitute   ¼ cup red and green
3 tablespoons water (omit   chopped bell pepper
    if substitute is used)   Optional: ½ teaspoon
    Salt and pepper   minced fresh garlic
8-ounce can plain tomato   Chili powder to taste
    sauce

Spray a nonstick skillet with cooking spray. Heat over moderate heat. When hot, add eggs beaten with water. Season to taste with salt and pepper. Cook undisturbed until eggs begin to set. Then gently lift edges of egg with a spatula allowing uncooked portion to run beneath. Continue cooking and lifting until eggs are soft-set with a moist creamy surface. Do not overcook. With spatula, gently fold omelet over on itself, then roll out of the skillet on to a heated plate. Cut in half and keep warm.

Put remaining ingredients into same skillet. Simmer uncovered 2 minutes until sauce is bubbling and thick. Pour over omelet halves and serve immediately.

Each portion (½ of the recipe) provides: 2 PR, 1 VEG

VARIATIONS

Mexican Cheese Omelet

Cook eggs as for Western omelet. Just before omelet is ready to be turned out of pan, sprinkle with 4 tablespoons shredded extra-sharp Cheddar or American-type diet cheese. Season the sauce with a pinch of cumin and oregano, if desired.

Each portion (½ of the recipe) provides: 3 PR, 1 VEG

Italian Omelet

Follow directions for Western Omelet, but omit chili powder. Season sauce with a dash of red pepper and oregano or mixed Italian seasonings.

Each portion (½ of the recipe) provides: 2 PR, 1 VEG

Italian Pizza Omelet

Follow Italian omelet directions, but just before turning omelet out of pan, sprinkle with 4 tablespoons of shredded part-skim mozzarella cheese.

Each portion (½ of the recipe) provides: 3 PR, 1 VEG

Yogurt Omelet   Serves 4

6 eggs (or equivalent egg   ½ cup plain low-fat yogurt
    substitute)   Salt, pepper, to taste

Beat ingredients together in a bowl. Spray a nonstick skillet
with cooking spray. Cook egg mixture in skillet gently over
low heat, lifting the edges and letting the liquid portion run
beneath to set.

Each portion (¼ of the recipe) provides: 1½ PR

Creole Omelet   Serves 2

2 ripe tomatoes, peeled   ¼ teaspoon dried oregano
    and chopped   Salt and pepper
¼ cup each, chopped green   4 eggs, lightly beaten (or
    bell pepper and celery   equivalent no-
2 tablespoons chopped   cholesterol egg
    onion   substitute)
¼ cup water

Combine vegetables, water, and oregano in a saucepan.
Cover and simmer 20 minutes, stirring occasionally. (Add
water, if needed.) Season to taste with salt and pepper.

Meanwhile, prepare a 2-serving omelet: Spray a nonstick
skillet with cooking spray. Heat over high heat. When skillet is hot, add the eggs. As eggs begin to set, lift the edges
gently, permitting unset portion to run beneath. Roll
cooked omelet onto a heated plate; top with vegetable
sauce. Cut in half to make 2 servings.

Each portion (½ of recipe) provides: 2 PR, 1 VEG

Fruit Omelet

Serves 2

½ cup cubed unpeeled red
    apple
¼ cup seedless green
    grapes
4 eggs, beaten (or
    equivalent no-

    cholesterol egg
    substitute)
4 ounces Cheddar-style
    "diet" cheese,
    shredded

Combine fruits at room temperature. Coat a 9-inch non-stick skillet with cooking spray. Heat skillet; when hot add eggs. As eggs begin to set, gently lift the edges allowing unset portion to run beneath. Sprinkle with cheese, then top with fruit. With a spatula, carefully fold omelet over. Turn omelet out of skillet onto an oven-proof dish. Place in a preheated 350-degree oven for 10 minutes until fruit is just warmed through and cheese is melted.

Each portion (½ of recipe) provides: 1 PR, 1 FR

Lean Blintzes

Serves 6

¾ cup flour
1 teaspoon butter-flavored
    salt
½ cup each skim milk and
    water
3 eggs plus 1 egg white

Filling
3 cups low-fat cottage
    cheese
1 egg yolk (or 2
    tablespoons no-
    cholesterol egg
    substitute)
½ teaspoon butter-flavored
    salt
¼ teaspoon grated lemon
    rind

Combine flour and butter-flavored salt. Gradually but thoroughly stir in the milk and water. Add eggs; beat smooth.

(continued)

LEAN BLINTZES, CONTINUED

Spray a 6-inch nonstick skillet with cooking spray. Pour about 2 tablespoons batter into pan. Tip and roll pan so that batter covers the bottom of skillet. Cook approximately 1 minute, until top of blintz dries. Turn blintz out of pan onto a towel, browned side down. Repeat until all batter is used.

Blend filling ingredients thoroughly. Place a spoonful of filling on each blintz. Fold in sides, then roll to make an envelope. At serving time, reheat in oven. Makes 18 blintzes. (Serve topped with Fresh Strawberry Spread [recipe p. 117], if desired.)

> **Each portion (3 blintzes) provides: 1 ST, 4 PR**
> *Toppings:* Refer to the 35-Plus Diet Food Lists to calculate additional ingredients. Limit Fresh Strawberry Spread to 1 tablespoon.

High-Fiber High-Protein French Toast   Serves 1

1 egg (or equivalent egg substitute)	salt (or butter-flavored salt)
1 tablespoon water	2 slices calorie-reduced bread (preferably high-fiber)
Optional: few drops vanilla extract, pinch of ground cinnamon, and	

Fork-blend the egg, water, and flavorings in a small shallow bowl. Soak bread in the mixture 3 to 5 minutes, turning slices, until all the liquid is absorbed.

Heat a nonstick skillet, sprayed with cooking spray, over medium heat. Cook bread slices, turning once until both sides are golden.

> **Each portion (one recipe) provides: 1 PR, 1 ST**

How about a sandwich for breakfast? These toaster-easy choices feature calorie-reduced bread and calcium-rich "light" cheeses topped with fruit instead of sugary jam or jelly. You can substitute any favorite fruit: sliced peach, apricot, apple, pear, or raisins.

Light Cream Cheese and Berries on Toast   Serves 1

2 slices light (calorie-reduced) bread, white or wheat, lightly toasted
1 ounce (2 tablespoons) light cream cheese or Neufchâtel cheese or Yogurt Cheese (recipe p. 201)

3 or 4 fresh strawberries, washed, hulled and thinly sliced
Optional: dash of ground cinnamon, low-calorie sweetener to taste

Spread 1 slice of toast with half of the light cream cheese and arrange the berries on top. Add a dash of cinnamon and low-calorie sweetener, if desired. Spread the other slice with remaining cream cheese and place over berries; cut sandwich into triangles to serve.

VARIATIONS

Substitute other fresh or partially thawed berries for the strawberries: blueberries or raspberries, for example, or thinly sliced fresh nectarines, grapes, or peeled peaches. Another good combination with the light cream cheese is ½ seedless orange, thinly sliced, 1 teaspoon raisins, and a pinch of pie spice.

Each portion (1 sandwich) provides: 1 PR, 1 ST, ½ FR

Farmer Cheese and Apple
Breakfast Sandwiches   Serves 1

2 slices light (calorie-
    reduced) bread, white
    or wheat, lightly
    toasted
2 tablespoons fresh soft
    farmer cheese (or dry
    cottage cheese)

¼ unpared red or yellow
    eating apple, cored
    and thinly sliced
Optional: pinch of pie spice
    and low-calorie
    sweetener to taste

Spread 1 slice of toast with half of the farmer cheese and
arrange the sliced apple on top. Add a shake of spice and
sweetener, if desired. Spread the other slice of toast with
remaining light cheese and place over fruit; cut sandwich
into triangles to serve.

Each portion (1 sandwich) provides: 1 PR, 1 ST, ¼ FR

Big Apple Bagel Thins and Cheese   Serves 1

2 thin slices (one-half
    regular size) whole
    wheat bagel, lightly
    toasted
2 tablespoons fresh soft
    farmer cheese (or dry
    cottage cheese)

¼ unpared red or yellow
    eating apple, cored
    and thinly sliced
Optional: pinch of pie spice
    and low-calorie
    sweetener to taste

Use fresh soft bagels, if possible. Slice each bagel into 4
thin slices; use 2 of the slices (half of a bagel) for each
serving. Toast bagel slices lightly.

    Spread 1 slice of toasted bagel thin with half of the
farmer cheese and arrange apple slices on top. Add a shake
of spice and sweetener, if desired. Spread the other slice of

toast with remaining light cheese and place over fruit; cut sandwich into triangles to serve.

Each portion (1 recipe) provides: 1 PR, 1 ST, ¼ FR

Pineapple-Cheese Danish Pita Pockets

Serves 1

1 whole wheat mini (1-ounce) pita bread
⅓ cup low-fat cottage cheese

2 tablespoons well drained, juice-packed crushed pineapple
Optional: ground cinnamon and low-calorie sweetener to taste

Toast the pita bread lightly. To serve, slice each pita bread in half to form 2 half moons. Combine remaining ingredients, mixing lightly, and divide between pita halves.

Each portion (1 sandwich) provides: 1 PR, 1 ST, ¼ FR

Cheese Danish and Spiced Pineapple on Crispbread

Serves 1

Tastes like a Danish pastry!

2 high-fiber crispbread crackers
1 ounce (2 tablespoons) light cream cheese or Neufchâtel cheese

1 tablespoon well drained juice-packed crushed pineapple
Optional: pinch of ground cinnamon and low-calorie sweetener

Spread each crispbread cracker with half of the light cream cheese and top with half of the crushed pineapple. Add a shake of cinnamon and low-calorie sweetener to each, if desired. Each portion (1 recipe) provides 1 PR, 1 ST, ½ FR

Berry Breakfast Cheese 'n' Crispbread   Serves 1

⅓ cup low-fat cottage
    cheese
Optional: a few drops
    vanilla extract
2 high-fiber crispbread
    crackers

¼ cup fresh blueberries,
    sliced strawberries,
    peaches, or nectarines
Optional: ground
    cinnamon, low-calorie
    sweetener to taste

Mix cottage cheese with vanilla, if desired. Spread each crispbread cracker with half of the cottage cheese and arrange fruit on top of each. Sprinkle lightly with cinnamon and sweetener, if desired.

Each portion (1 sandwich) provides: 1 PR, 1 ST, ½ FR

Cheese and Orange Spread   Serves 4
(2 tablespoons per serving)

8 ounces "light" (calorie-
    reduced) cream cheese
    or fresh (soft) farmer
    cheese

4 tablespoons orange juice
    concentrate

For easiest mixing, allow both ingredients to reach room temperature, then beat together until fluffy. Store in the refrigerator. (May be sweetened with sugar substitute and spiced with a pinch of cinnamon to taste, if desired.)

Each portion (2 tablespoons) provides: 1 PR

Blueberry Jam   Makes 10 8-ounce jars

5 pints fresh blueberries
1 envelope plain gelatin

6-ounce can apple juice
    concentrate, thawed,
    divided
2 tablespoons lemon juice

Puree blueberries in food processor or blender, 1 or 2 pints at a time; set aside. Sprinkle the gelatin on half the apple juice concentrate in a small pan or microwave dish. While gelatin is softening, combine remaining apple juice concentrate with lemon juice.

When the gelatin is soft, heat gently until melted. Combine melted gelatin, fruit juice, and pureed blueberries; mix well. Spoon into 8-ounce jelly jars; label and store in refrigerator freezer. Keep refrigerated.

VARIATION

Blackberry Jam

For best results, combine fresh blackberries with blueberries to minimize the seediness of the blackberries. Follow preceding recipe, using 3 pints blueberries and 4 small half-pint boxes of fresh blackberries.

Limit servings to 1 tablespoon per day.

Fresh Strawberry Spread

Makes 3 8-ounce jars

1 pint fresh strawberries
1 package (4-serving)
   sugar-free strawberry
   gelatin

1 cup boiling water

Wash, hull, and mash the berries well. Stir the gelatin into boiling water until completely dissolved, then combine with mashed berries. Refrigerate (stir once or twice) until set. Spoon into covered jelly jars and store in the refrigerator.

Limit servings to 1 tablespoon per day.

Speedy Strawberry Syrup   Makes 1 cup

½ cup low-sugar or   ½ cup water
   sugarless strawberry   Optional: 3 packets low-
   jam or preserves (or   calorie sweetener
   any favorite flavor)

Combine jam and water in a saucepan. Cook and stir over
low heat until simmering. Remove from heat and stir in
sugar substitute, if desired. Serve with pancakes or French
toast.

Limit servings to 1 tablespoon per day.

12 Lunch and Supper

These recipes are apportioned for lunch or light supper. In many instances, the size of each portion can be doubled to provide you with an entree suitable for your main meal. Check allowances carefully, particularly for carbohydrate (ST) content to be sure that a larger portion does not exceed your carbohydrate allowance.

Mideastern Sloppy Joes

Serves 4

1 pound fat-trimmed lean beef round, ground
1½ cups chopped onion
¾ cup each chopped celery and bell pepper
8 ounces plain tomato sauce

4 tablespoons each lemon juice and minced fresh parsley
1 tablespoon cumin seeds Garlic salt, pepper, to taste
4 whole wheat mini 1-ounce pita breads with sesame seeds

Spray a large nonstick skillet or electric frying pan with cooking spray. Spread the beef in a shallow layer and brown over high heat. When underside is done, break the meat into chunks and turn it to brown evenly. Discard any melted fat from pan. Stir in the onion; cook and stir just until onion begins to brown. Stir in celery, bell pepper, and tomato sauce. Add lemon juice, parsley, and seasonings.

Toast the pita breads lightly. To serve, slice each pita pocket partially around the border, then open to form a pocket. Spoon in the spicy beef mixture and serve immediately.

Each portion (¼ of the recipe) provides: 3 PR, 1 ST, 1 VEG

Aegean Beefy Pita Pockets   Serves 4

4 broiled hamburgers
8-ounce can stewed
    tomatoes
1 onion, chopped
2 tablespoons chopped
    fresh (or 2 teaspoons
    dried) mint or
    oregano

Dash each ground
    cinnamon and
    nutmeg
4 (1-ounce) mini pita
    breads
12 dill pickle slices
4 ounces crumbled feta
    (or shredded Romano)
    cheese

Break up hamburgers; combine in a saucepan with tomatoes, onion, herbs, and spices. Simmer until hamburger is heated through.

Split pita breads around edges and open to form pockets. Spoon the hot mixture into the pockets; add pickles and cheese.

Each portion (¼ of recipe) provides: 4 PR, 1 ST

Barbecue in a Pita Pocket   Serves 4

1½ cups plain or seasoned
    tomato juice
1 tablespoon cider
    vinegar
6 tablespoons
    unsweetened
    pineapple (or apple)
    juice
2 tablespoons
    Worcestershire sauce
1 tablespoon minced
    onion
1 clove garlic, minced

½ teaspoon celery seed
¼ teaspoon paprika
Pinch of ground cloves
½ to 1 teaspoon chili
    powder (or more to
    taste)
2 cups fat-trimmed, lean
    roast beef or pork,
    minced or thinly
    sliced
Optional: 2 to 3 packets
    low-calorie sweetener
4 mini pita breads

Combine tomato juice, vinegar, fruit juice, Worcestershire sauce, and all seasonings in a saucepan. Simmer uncovered 6 to 8 minutes, until sauce is thick. Stir in meat and heat through. Remove from heat and stir in low-calorie sweetener, if desired. Spoon meat and sauce mixture over slightly toasted, small pita breads, split to form pockets.

Each portion (¼ of the recipe) provides: 3 PR, 1 ST

Sloppy Joe Spaghetti Squash

Serves 4

1 medium spaghetti squash	8-ounce can plain tomato sauce
1 cup water	12 ounces mixed vegetable juice
1 pound extra-lean ground beef	1 cup chopped bell pepper
1 teaspoon each oregano, basil, garlic salt, and pepper to taste	4-ounce can mushrooms, undrained
Optional: pinch of red pepper flakes	Optional: 4 tablespoons grated Romano cheese
16-ounce can stewed tomatoes	

Puncture the spaghetti squash in several places with a skewer. Put the squash in a shallow roasting pan, add water, and bake it uncovered in a preheated 350-degree oven about 45 minutes.

While squash is baking, prepare the sauce. Coat a large nonstick skillet or electric frypan with cooking spray. Spread the ground meat in a shallow layer; sprinkle it with herbs and seasonings. Brown the meat with no fat added over moderate heat. When the underside is brown, break the meat into chunks and turn the chunks over to brown evenly. Drain and discard fat from pan. Stir in remaining

(continued)

ingredients (except cheese). Cover and simmer 5 minutes. Uncover and simmer until sauce is thick and reduced, about 20 to 25 minutes more.

Remove the squash from the oven and slice it in half; scrape out and discard the seeds. Scrape out the yellow strands and fluff with the tines of a fork to form a vegetable spaghetti.

To serve, spoon the meat sauce over the spaghetti squash (and sprinkle with grated cheese if desired).

Each portion (¼ of the recipe) provides: 3½ PR, 1 VEG

One-Step Lazy Lasagna   Serves 8

This version contains more protein than pasta, and the lasagna noodles need no precooking.

7 ounces uncooked high-protein lasagna noodles
½ cup boiling water
4 cups uncreamed, pot-style cottage cheese
2 beaten eggs (or ½ cup no-cholesterol substitute)
4 tablespoons minced fresh parsley
4 tablespoons minced chives (or onion)
1 teaspoon each dried oregano and basil

Dash each garlic salt and ground nutmeg
3½ cups canned tomatoes in puree, divided
12 thin slices (6 ounces) part-skim mozzarella cheese
¾ pound extra lean ground beef or veal
Dash of coarse pepper
3 tablespoons each Italian-seasoned bread crumbs and grated Romano cheese

Arrange half of the uncooked noodles in a single layer in the bottom of a nonstick rectangular 9 x 13-inch baking pan; break up the noodles to fit. Pour on the boiling water. Set aside.

Stir the cottage cheese with the eggs, parsley, chives, oregano, basil, garlic salt, and nutmeg. Spread the mixture evenly over the layer of dry noodles. Cover with remaining noodles, arranged in a single layer. Pour on 3 cups of tomatoes, reserving ½ cup of the puree. Add the mozzarella in a single layer and cover with remaining tomato puree.

Season the ground meat to taste with garlic salt and pepper. Arrange the meat mixture in chunks on top. Sprinkle with bread crumbs and Romano.

Cover the pan with foil and bake in a preheated 350-degree oven for 1 hour. Uncover and bake an additional 30 to 45 minutes, until topping is crusty. Let stand at room temperature 15 minutes before cutting. Makes 8 servings.

Each portion (⅛ of the recipe) provides: 3 PR, 1 ST

Frozen Dinners: Leftover lasagna can be divided into single servings, wrapped, labeled, and frozen. Reheat in oven or microwave.

VARIATION

Veal-Eggplant-Cheese Casserole

Substitute 1 large eggplant, thinly sliced, for the lasagna noodles; omit the boiling water. Use ground veal in place of beef. Reduce baking time to 1½ hours.

Each portion (⅛ of the recipe) provides: 3 PR, ¼ VEG

Beef Fajitas   Serves 4

Fajitas are soft flour tortillas filled with marinated lean beef and spicy toppings

2 cups leftover roast beef
   (lean only), thinly
   sliced
2 tablespoons lime (or
   lemon) juice
1 garlic clove, minced
4 flour tortillas
4 slices ripe tomato
8 thin dill pickle slices

Optional: chili sauce or
   Tabasco
4 tablespoons each
   chopped onion, minced
   cilantro leaves (or
   parsley), plain low-fat
   yogurt (instead of sour
   cream)

Combine meat in a plastic bag with lime juice and garlic. Marinate 30 minutes at room temperature or several hours in the refrigerator.

Wrap tortillas in foil and warm them in a 350-degree oven 6 to 8 minutes. Leave them wrapped in foil.

Prepare and assemble remaining ingredients. Gently heat beef in its marinade.

For each serving, combine sliced beef on a warm tortilla and garnish with a slice of tomato, pickle, and a tablespoon each of chopped onion, cilantro, chili sauce, yogurt. Fold up and eat with fingers.

Each portion (¼ of the recipe) provides: 3 PR, 1 ST

VARIATION

Fajita Pitas

Replace the flour tortillas with small 1-ounce pita breads, lightly toasted. Split each pita at the edge to form a pocket and divide cooked lean beef and other ingredients among them.

Each portion (¼ of the recipe) provides: 3 PR, 1 ST

Skinny Skillet Chili   Serves 4

1 pound fat-trimmed
    ground beef round
2 cups canned kidney
    beans, drained
16-ounce can tomatoes
8-ounce can plain tomato
    sauce

2 onions, chopped
1 bell pepper, seeded and
    chopped
1 or 2 cloves garlic,
    minced
1 tablespoon chili powder
    (or more, to taste)

Brown beef in a nonstick skillet with no fat added. Break into chunks and turn to brown evenly. Drain and discard fat from pan.

Stir in all remaining ingredients. Cover and simmer 20 minutes. Uncover and continue cooking until thickened.

Each portion (¼ of the recipe) provides: 3 PR, 1 ST

Budget Veal Cutlet   Serves 4

1 pound fat-trimmed
    ground veal
1 egg, beaten (or
    equivalent no-
    cholesterol egg
    substitute)
  Grated peel of 1 lemon

¼ teaspoon grated nutmeg
  Salt (or onion salt),
    pepper, to taste
6 tablespoons Italian-
    seasoned bread
    crumbs

Spray a large nonstick griddle or skillet with cooking spray. Combine ingredients, except bread crumbs, and mix lightly.

Sprinkle half the bread crumbs on a shallow plate. Shape one quarter of meat mixture into a flat "cutlet" and press into the crumbs, lightly coating both sides. Place cutlet on griddle, and make 3 more with remaining meat mixture and bread crumbs.

(continued)

BUDGET VEAL CUTLET, CONTINUED

Brown over moderate heat. Turn cutlets to brown other side evenly. Cook about 2 to 3 minutes per side.

Each portion (¼ of the recipe) provides: 3 PR, ¼ ST

VARIATION

Veal Cutlets Parmigiana

Follow preceding recipe. Top each serving with ½ cup oregano-seasoned tomato sauce and a 1-ounce slice of part-skim mozzarella cheese.

Each portion (¼ of the recipe) provides: 4 PR, ¼ ST

Vealburgers Paprikash   Serves 4

1 pound fat-trimmed
    ground veal
½ cup plain low-fat yogurt
2 tablespoons
    Worcestershire sauce

3 tablespoons chopped (or
    1 tablespoon dried)
    onion flakes
1 tablespoon paprika
    Garlic salt, pepper, to
      taste
2 cups sliced mushrooms

Combine ingredients, except mushrooms. Shape into 4 "cutlets." Arrange on a baking tray in a single layer; surround with mushrooms. Bake in preheated 475-degree oven, 8 to 10 minutes each side.

Each portion (¼ of the recipe) provides: 3 PR, 1 VEG

Lemon Vealburgers with Capers   Serves 8

2 pounds ground veal
1 small onion, minced
1 egg (or no-cholesterol
    equivalent)

4 tablespoons seasoned
    bread crumbs
Coarse black pepper
8 teaspoons drained capers
Juice of 2 lemons

Lightly mix veal, onion, egg, and bread crumbs. Season
with pepper (but omit any salt). Take half of the meat mixture and shape it into 8 small patties. Flatten each patty
gently. Place a teaspoon of capers in the middle of each.
Sprinkle with more pepper and lemon juice.

Shape remaining meat mixture into 8 more patties. Arrange these on top of the first patties, so that the capers are
inside, and you have 8 stuffed patties. Gently press edges
of each patty together, sealing the stuffing inside. Brush
lightly with additional lemon juice. Broil or barbecue 3
inches from heat source about 4 to 5 minutes per side.

Each portion (⅛ of recipe) provides: 3 PR, ¼ ST

Quiche Lorraine   Serves 8

8 ounces sliced ham (or
    Canadian bacon)
6 eggs (or equivalent egg
    substitute)
1 cup skim milk
½ cup minced onion

1 tablespoon chopped
    chives
Dash each of nutmeg
    and pepper
10 ounces grated low-fat
    cheese

Coat a 9-inch pie pan with cooking spray and arrange ham
(or Canadian bacon) in dish. Beat eggs, add milk, onions,
chives, and seasonings. Mix well. Stir in grated cheese.
Pour mixture over ham or Canadian bacon.

Bake at 325 degrees for 35 to 45 minutes, or until a knife
inserted into the center comes out clean.

Each portion (⅛ of the recipe) provides: 3 PR

Polynesian Chicken Salad   Serves 4

2 cups (about 12 ounces)
   diced, cooked, white-
   meat chicken
2 tablespoons soy sauce
2 cups each diced celery,
   fresh (or juice-packed
   canned, drained)
   pineapple tidbits
½ cup canned water
   chestnuts, sliced and
   drained (or fresh
   sunchokes or jícama)

3 tablespoons each low-
   calorie mayonnaise,
   plain (or pineapple)
   low-fat yogurt,
   unsweetened
   pineapple juice (from
   canned pineapple, if
   you are using it)
Pinch of ground
   cinnamon
Lettuce

Stir chicken with soy sauce and marinate 15 to 20 minutes. Mix with remaining ingredients, except lettuce. Mound on beds of lettuce.

Each portion (¼ of the recipe) provides: 3 PR, 1 VEG

Oven Turkey Barbecue   Serves 6

2-pound turkey roast
1 tablespoon prepared
   mustard
½ cup each red wine vinegar,
   chili sauce, light beer,
   and tomato juice

Garlic salt, coarse
   pepper, to taste

Use turkey roast frozen or thawed. Combine remaining ingredients and pour over turkey. Roast uncovered at 350 degrees, about 1½ (thawed) to 2 hours (frozen), until a meat thermometer registers 175 degrees. Baste occasionally. (If roasting from frozen state, insert thermometer after cooking 1 hour.)

Each portion (⅙ of the recipe) provides: 3 PR

Mexican Turkey Salad

Serves 4

1 head iceberg lettuce, shredded

4 tablespoons minced onion

1 red (or green) bell pepper, diced

Optional: 1 fresh jalapeno pepper, chopped (or chili powder, to taste)

1 ripe tomato, cubed

Optional: 4 tablespoons chopped fresh cilantro (or parsley)

2 cups cubed cooked turkey roast

6 tablespoons low-calorie Italian salad dressing

2 teaspoons cumin seeds (or 1 teaspoon ground cumin)

4 ounces each shredded Cheddar-style diet cheese, broken tortilla chips

Toss vegetables and turkey with salad dressing. Sprinkle with cumin, cheese, and tortilla chips.

Each portion (¼ of recipe) provides: 4 PR, 1 ST

Seafood Fried Rice

Serves 6

2¾ cups water, divided

1 cup each uncooked long-grain rice and finely minced celery

2 eggs, beaten (or equivalent no-cholesterol substitute)

4 ounces lean boiled ham, cubed

1 onion, chopped

½ cup sliced mushrooms

6-ounce can small shrimp

6-ounce package crabmeat, defrosted

2 teaspoons ground ginger

3 scallions, sliced

Optional: light soy sauce

Heat 1¾ cups water to boiling; add rice and celery. Cover; simmer 20 to 25 minutes, stirring occasionally, until liquid is absorbed.

Meanwhile, spray a large nonstick skillet with cooking

(continued)

SEAFOOD FRIED RICE, CONTINUED

spray; add eggs. Heat gently until partly set; then break up
with a fork. Remove eggs from pan and set aside.

Clean skillet. Add ham. Cook with no fat added, turning
occasionally, until lightly browned. Remove ham and set
aside.

Add ¼ cup water to skillet. Add onion; cook, stirring
occasionally, until water evaporates and onion is golden.
Add mushrooms, undrained shrimp, crabmeat, cooked
rice-celery mixture, eggs, ginger, and ham. Cook and stir
over medium heat until most liquid in pan evaporates. Stir
in scallions at last minute. Serve with soy sauce, if desired.

Each portion (⅙ of the recipe) provides: 3 PR, 1 ST

Fish Fu Yung   Serves 4

8 beaten eggs (or 2 cups
  no-cholesterol egg
  substitute)
1 cup cooked seafood
  (flaked fish, tiny
  shelled shrimp,
  shredded crabmeat or
  lobster, or a mixture)
⅛ cup each diagonally
  sliced celery, thinly
  sliced scallions, bean
  sprouts (or equivalent
  mixed drained
  Oriental vegetables)

2 tablespoons chopped
  fresh cilantro (or
  parsley) leaves
Optional: ½ teaspoon
  chopped fresh anise
  (or fennel) seeds
Fu Yung Sauce (see page
  188)

Spray a large nonstick skillet or round electric frying pan
with cooking spray; preheat moderately. Add the beaten
eggs or thawed egg substitute. Cook undisturbed until
edges of egg mixture appear set, then lift gently with a
spatula to permit some of the uncooked egg to run under-
neath.

Sprinkle remaining ingredients, except sauce, on top. Lower heat; cover pan, and cook over low heat while you make the sauce. Keep pan covered until ready to serve. Cut the Fu Yung into 4 wedges, and top each serving with sauce.

Each portion (¼ of the recipe) provides: 3 PR, 1 VEG

VARIATIONS

In each of the following recipes, cook according to general directions under Fish Fu Yung.

Vegetable Fu Yung

8 beaten eggs (or 2 cups no-cholesterol egg substitute)
½ cup each sliced fresh mushrooms, raw broccoli florets, cubed raw zucchini, chopped sweet onion

¼ cup each diagonally sliced celery, chopped sweet bell pepper
2 tablespoons chopped fresh cilantro (or parsley) leaves
Fu Yung Sauce (see page 188)

Follow the preceding directions.

Each portion (¼ of the recipe) provides: 2 PR, 1 VEG

Mushroom-Beef Fu Yung

8 beaten eggs (or 2 cups no-cholesterol egg substitute)
1 cup thinly sliced rare cooked steak or leftover roast beef (lean only)

1 cup sliced fresh mushrooms
½ cup sliced sweet onion
2 tablespoons sesame seeds
Fu Yung Sauce (see page 188)

Follow preceding directions. Cut into wedges and serve with Fu Yung Sauce.

Each portion (¼ of the recipe) provides: 3 PR, ½ VEG

(continued)

VARIATIONS FOR FISH FU YUNG, CONTINUED

Smoked Turkey Fu Yung

8 beaten eggs (or 2 cups
    no-cholesterol egg
    substitute)
1 cup diced smoked turkey
    (or lean cooked ham)
½ cup each diced red and
    green bell pepper,
    drained juice-packed
    canned pineapple
    tidbits (reserve juice)

¼ cup each diagonally
    sliced celery, sliced
    scallions
Fu Yung Sauce (see page
    188)

Note: Follow preceding directions. In Fu Yung Sauce, use reserved juice from pineapple in place of part of the broth or other liquid.

Each portion (¼ of the recipe) provides: 3 PR, 1 VEG, ¼ FR

Marinated Sardines   Serves 4 for lunch, 8 for appetizers

7 ounces brine-packed
    sardines
1 cup white vinegar

1 tablespoon each dill seed
    and lemon juice
Optional: fresh dill leaves

Use sardines packed in brine rather than in oil; drain well and set aside.

Heat vinegar to boiling; stir in dill seed and lemon juice. Pour mixture over sardines. When cool, refrigerate several hours or overnight. Drain well and garnish with fresh dill leaves, if you are using them. Serve on rye crackers, if desired.

For lunch, each portion (¼ of recipe) provides: 1 PR
For appetizers, each portion (⅛ of recipe) provides: ½ PR
With 3 rye crackers, add: 1 ST

Calories and Calcium in Sardines

3½ ounces	calories	calcium in mg
in tomato sauce	196	446
in mustard sauce	194	301
in oil, drained	203	434
in brine	194	301

Sardines are named for the Island of Sardinia, off the west coast of Italy. What other food can you think of where you actually eat the bones! Because these tiny fish have a skeleton as fine as a spiderweb, the bones are consumed along with the fish. As a result, a tiny can of sardines has more calcium than a big glass of milk.

Sauced Sardines
Serves 2 for lunch, 4 for appetizers

8 ounces sardines in tomato
    sauce
4 tablespoons catsup
1 tablespoon each lemon
    juice and prepared
    horseradish

Carefully remove sardines from their sauce. Combine the tomato sauce with remaining ingredients. Spoon the cocktail sauce into little cups for dipping. Arrange sardines on lettuce and garnish with cherry tomatoes, pepper rings, and cucumber slices, if desired.

    For lunch, each portion (½ of the recipe) provides: 1 PR
    For appetizers, each portion (¼ of the recipe) provides: ½ PR

13 Salads and Salad Dressings

The first three recipes are for hearty, meal-sized salads. You will find additional meal-sized salad recipes under the Lunch and Supper, Main Course, and Pasta sections.

Nicoise-style Tuna Salad

Serves 2

10 ounces thawed (or fresh) uncooked green beans
7-ounce can water-packed solid white tuna
1 tomato, sliced
¼ of a red onion, thinly sliced
Optional: ¼ of a red (or green) bell pepper, sliced
3 ripe olives, pitted and sliced

4 tablespoons olive liquid (from olive container)
2 tablespoons wine vinegar
½ teaspoon Worcestershire sauce
⅛ teaspoon instant garlic
Salt and freshly ground pepper
Optional: Romaine lettuce

Combine ingredients, except lettuce. Refrigerate several hours, if possible. Serve on lettuce, if desired.

Each portion (½ of the recipe) provides: 2 PR, ½ VEG

Chicken Vegetable Salad   Serves 3

1 cup cooked, chilled (or
    canned, drained)
    sliced potatoes
10-ounce package frozen
    kitchen-cut green
    beans
½ cup fresh (or frozen) red
    and green diced bell
    pepper
¼ cup frozen chives (or
    fresh chopped onion
    or scallion)
2-ounce can sliced
    mushrooms, chilled
10 pitted black olives,
    sliced
3 tablespoons each olive
    liquid (from olive
    container) and lemon
    juice (or cider vinegar)

Optional: 2 tablespoons
    minced fresh parsley
2 teaspoons fresh (or half-
    teaspoon dried) thyme
1 teaspoon each fresh
    basil and oregano (or
    1 teaspoon dried
    Italian herbs)
Garlic salt, pepper, to
    taste
1 cup diced cooked white-
    meat chicken
1 large ripe tomato, cut in
    cubes (or small cherry
    tomatoes)

Frozen vegetables should be slightly thawed and drained; do not cook.

Place potatoes in a large plastic bowl with a tight-fitting lid. Break up and add green beans, bell pepper, and chives. Stir in undrained mushrooms, olives, olive liquid, lemon juice, herbs, and seasonings. Mix lightly. Add chicken and tomato last. Cover tightly and chill.

Each portion (⅓ of the recipe) provides: 1½ PR, 2 VEG, ⅓ ST

Curried Chicken Salad Veronica   Serves 1

½ cup diced cooked white meat chicken

2 teaspoons minced fresh tarragon leaves (or parsley)

¼ cup green grapes, halved

1 tablespoon snipped chives (or sliced scallions)

¼ teaspoon curry powder
Salt (or seasoned salt), pepper, to taste

2 cups torn lettuce

1 tablespoon each low-calorie mayonnaise and plain low-fat yogurt

Optional: pinch of cumin seeds

Arrange chicken, grapes, and chives on top of lettuce. Stir remaining ingredients together and spoon over salad.

Each portion (1 recipe) provides: 2 PR, 2 VEG, 1 FR

Spiced Chickpeas   Serves 6

1 cup dried chickpeas (ceci or garbanzo beans)

½ cup red (or green) bell pepper, diced

1 cup chopped onions

1 to 2 teaspoons curry powder (to taste)

1 clove garlic, minced

2 teaspoons whole cumin seeds

Salt or lemon pepper (to taste)

10 ounces frozen green peas

1½ cups water

1½ cups fat-skimmed chicken broth (or additional water)

Cover chickpeas with water and soak overnight, or boil 2 minutes and let soak 1 hour.

Combine onions, garlic, and cumin seeds in a large non-stick skillet or electric frying pan that has been generously coated with cooking spray. Cook and stir uncovered until moisture evaporates and onions begin to brown. Add drained chickpeas and 3 cups liquid (water or broth or a mixture). Stir in remaining ingredients except peas. Cover and simmer until chickpeas are tender, about 2 hours.

Add green peas and cook uncovered just until peas are thawed and heated through, 6 to 8 minutes. Makes 6 servings.

Each portion (⅙ of the recipe) provides: 1 ST

Italian Bean Salad   Serves 8

16-ounce can each cut green beans and cut wax beans (yellow string beans)
6 tablespoons liquid from canned green beans
1 small red (or yellow) onion, very thinly sliced

½ cup diced sweet red pepper, fresh or canned
4 tablespoons lemon juice (or cider vinegar)
1 teaspoon dried oregano
Optional: 1 clove garlic, finely minced
Salt (or garlic salt), coarse pepper, to taste

Drain beans, reserving 6 tablespoons of liquid. Combine all ingredients in a glass bowl. Cover and refrigerate 2 hours or more before serving.

Each portion (⅛ of the recipe) provides: 1 VEG

Quick Bean Salad   Serves 2

8-ounce can green or yellow beans, drained

1 tablespoon dried onions
Shake of dried oregano

Combine ingredients and refrigerate until dinnertime.

Each portion (½ of the recipe) provides: 1 VEG

Broccoli Horseradish Salad   Serves 2

2 cups sliced raw broccoli   2 teaspoons prepared white
2 tablespoons low-calorie   horseradish
    mayonnaise   Lemon pepper to taste

To prepare broccoli, trim and slice away tough outer layer
of stalks. Slice inner stalks into thin chips. Break up heads
into florets. Rinse in cold water; drain well and combine
with remaining ingredients.

Each portion (½ of the recipe) provides: 2 VEG

Chilled and Ready Salad   Serves 4 (approximate)

1 head lettuce   1 bell pepper
1 small red onion   1 cup cherry tomatoes
1 small cucumber

Tear lettuce into bite-size pieces; slice onion thin and separate into rings. Slice cucumber and dice pepper. Combine
all ingredients in a big plastic bag. Refrigerate without
washing.

At dinnertime, take out as much salad as you need and
rinse in ice-cold water. Drain well and place in single salad
bowls. Top each serving with your favorite low-calorie
dressing.

Each portion (about ¼ of the recipe) provides: 2 VEG

Cucumber-Tomato Relish   Serves 8

2 ripe tomatoes, peeled and
    cubed
1 medium cucumber, pared
    and chopped
3 tablespoons each
    chopped onions (or
    sliced scallions) and
    fresh minced parsley
1 teaspoon each fresh (or ¼
    teaspoon each dried)
    basil, thyme, and
    oregano

4 tablespoons olive liquid
    (from container of
    olives)
3 tablespoons cider vinegar
    Salt (or garlic salt), coarse
    pepper, to taste
Optional: 1 teaspoon
    prepared mustard

Combine vegetables and herbs in a bowl. Combine remaining ingredients and mix well; pour over vegetables. Cover and refrigerate several hours to allow flavors to blend.

Each portion (⅛ of the recipe) provides: ¼ VEG

Here are three recipes for basic low-fat mayonnaise dressings.

High-Protein Mayonnaise   Makes about 1½ cups

1 hard-cooked egg,
    chopped
⅛ teaspoon celery salt
1 to 3 packets low-calorie
    sweetener (optional)

1 tablespoon skim milk
½ teaspoon paprika
1 cup low-fat cottage
    cheese
1 tablespoon minced onion
2 tablespoons lemon juice

Blend smooth in blender. Keep refrigerated in a covered jar.

Each portion (2 tablespoons) provides: ¼ PR

Slim and Tangy
Mayonnaise Dressing

Makes about 1⅓ cups

½ cup plain low-fat
    mayonnaise
⅓ cup plain low-fat yogurt
¼ cup each: cider vinegar,
    water

Garlic, onion or celery
    salt, coarse pepper,
    other seasonings, to
    taste

With a wire whisk, gently fold ingredients together until
smooth. Add more water if a thinner dressing is desired.

    **Each portion (2 tablespoons) provides a small fraction of your
    allowance of milk products**

Mayogurt

Makes about 1¼ cups

Use this recipe as the base for variations below.

1 cup plain low-fat yogurt
2 hard-cooked eggs
2 tablespoons lemon juice

1 teaspoon celery salt
½ teaspoon each dry
    mustard and sugar

Combine ingredients in a blender or food processor, using
the steel blade. Process until smooth.

    **Each portion (2 tablespoons) provides a small fraction of your
    ML and PR allowances**

VARIATIONS

Creamy Italian Herb

Add 1 or 2 cloves minced garlic, 1 teaspoon each dried
basil and oregano (or 1 tablespoon each of the fresh herbs).

Creamy Romano

Prepare Creamy Italian Herb; add 4 tablespoons grated
sharp Romano cheese.

Light and Creamy Russian

Add ½ cup catsup or chili sauce.

Light and Creamy Thousand Island

Stir in ⅓ cup chili sauce and ¼ cup dill pickle relish.

Green Goddess

Add ½ cup finely chopped fresh parsley and 4 table-spoons minced chives or scallions.

Creamy Garlic

Add 3 to 4 cloves minced garlic or 2 teaspoons dried garlic.

Creamy Cucumber

Remove the seeds from half of a medium peeled cucumber and puree the cucumber in a food processor or blender. Fold the puree into the other ingredients.

Creamy Horseradish

Add 3 to 4 tablespoons (to taste) well-drained prepared white horseradish.

Curry Dressing

Add 2 to 3 teaspoons curry powder and 1 teaspoon whole cumin seeds (or to taste).

Poppy Seed Dressing

Add 1 to 2 tablespoons poppy seeds.

Dill Dressing (for coleslaw, potato, or macaroni salad)

Follow recipe for Mayogurt, page 140, adding 4 tablespoons minced fresh dill leaves (or 2 tablespoons each dill seeds and minced parsley).

Buttermilk Dressing   Makes about 2 cups

1 package of dry buttermilk dressing	1 cup low-fat cottage cheese
	1 cup low-fat milk

Blend smooth in blender. Refrigerate in covered jar.
> Each portion (2 tablespoons) provides a small fraction of your ML and PR allowances

Devilish Yogurt Salad Dressing   Makes about 1 cup

1 cup plain low-fat yogurt	2 teaspoons lemon juice
1 tablespoon prepared mustard	1 clove garlic, minced
	Salt, coarse pepper, to taste

Gently fold ingredients together. Cover and store in the refrigerator. Great with pasta or potato salad.
> Each portion (2 tablespoons) provides: 1/8 ML

Slim Vinaigrette

Makes about ¾ cup

1 small (or ½ medium)
   onion, peeled
1 or 2 cloves garlic, peeled
⅓ cup boiling water
1 to 2 tablespoons each
   cider (or white)
   vinegar and lemon (or
   lime) juice

Salt, pepper, to taste
Optional: 1 teaspoon
   prepared mustard

Combine ingredients in blender. Cover; blend smooth. Chill in refrigerator. Shake before using.

Nutrients per portion (2 tablespoons) are negligible

Gazpacho Salad Dressing

Makes 2 cups

The ingredients of Spain's "salad soup" combine to make a zesty low-calorie dressing for tossed greens.

1 cup tomato juice
4 tablespoons olive
   packing liquid
1 onion, sliced
1 small red (or green)
   sweet pepper, cut up

½ cucumber, pared
½ cup parsley
2 cloves garlic
   Salt, coarse pepper, to
   taste

Combine ingredients in blender or food processor; cover and process smooth. Store in a covered jar. Shake dressing well before using. Spoon over chilled torn lettuce.

Nutrients per portion (2 tablespoons) are negligible

14 Lean Protein Main Courses: Meat, Poultry, and Seafood

These recipes are apportioned for the largest meal of the day. In most instances, the size of each portion can be halved to provide you with an entree suitable for lunch or a light supper.

Oven-Baked Beef Parmigiana

Serves 4

4 tablespoons Italian-
    seasoned bread crumbs
4 tablespoons grated
    Romano (or Parmesan
    cheese)
1 pound machine-
    tenderized beef round
    "minute steaks" (4
    steaks)

8-ounce can plain tomato
    sauce
8 ounces shredded part-
    skim mozzarella cheese
Pinch each dried
    oregano, basil, and
    garlic

Preheat oven to 475 degrees. Coat a shallow nonstick heavy baking dish with cooking spray. Combine the bread crumbs and Romano (or Parmesan) on a plate; press each steak into the mixture, lightly coating both sides. Arrange the steaks in a single layer on the baking dish. Bake uncovered, 8 to 10 minutes, until browned.

Pour tomato sauce over steaks. Arrange the mozzarella on top and sprinkle with herbs. Put the baking dish back in the oven and lower heat to 350 degrees. Bake 8 to 10 minutes more, until cheese and sauce are bubbling.

Each portion (¼ of the recipe) provides: 5 PR, ½ ST

Eggplant Parmesan

Serves 4

1 large eggplant	1 tablespoon minced
1½ pounds lean ground	onion
beef or veal	Salt and pepper to taste
12-ounce can tomato juice	8 ounces part-skim
1 tablespoon fresh	mozzarella cheese
minced basil	2 teaspoons grated
1 teaspoon oregano	Parmesan cheese
1 clove garlic, minced	

About half an hour before cooking, peel skin from eggplant and slice it. Sprinkle salt over it very lightly, then place it aside to drain.

Brown meat in sprayed pan, add tomato juice, basil, oregano, garlic, and onion. Add pepper, and salt if desired. Simmer until slightly thickened.

Coat a 2-quart casserole with cooking spray and layer, alternately, meat sauce, drained eggplant, and mozzarella. Finish with meat sauce and sprinkle Parmesan over the top. Bake at 350 degrees until eggplant is soft, about 35 to 45 minutes.

Each portion (¼ of the recipe) provides: 6 PR, 2 VEG

Italian-Style Swiss Steak

Serves 4

2 pounds fat-trimmed top	6 cups tomato juice
round steak	2 tablespoons lemon juice
½ cup each chopped onion,	1 clove garlic, minced
celery, and green bell	1 teaspoon dried oregano
pepper	

Coat a large nonstick skillet or electric frying pan with cooking spray. Heat over moderate flame. Brown steak quickly on both sides. Drain and discard any melted fat.

(continued)

Place the onion, celery, and peppers under steak. Add remaining ingredients. Cover and simmer over low heat until beef is very tender, 1 hour or more. Uncover and continue to simmer until liquid evaporates into a thick sauce.

VARIATION

Tex-Mex-Style Swiss Steak

Add 1 tablespoon chili powder and 2 teaspoons cumin seeds.

Each portion (¼ of the recipe) provides: 6 PR, 1½ VEG

Slimmer Swiss Steak   Serves 2

1 pound top round steak
½ cup each chopped onion
    and chopped celery
8-ounce can stewed
    tomatoes
4-ounce can mushroom
    stems and pieces,
    undrained

1 teaspoon dried savory (or
    sage and marjoram)
Optional: salt (or garlic
    salt), coarse pepper, to
    taste

Brown beef on both sides in a large nonstick skillet coated with cooking spray. Arrange the chopped onion and celery under steak. Add remaining ingredients on top. Cover and simmer until steak is tender, about 1 hour. Uncover and simmer until sauce is thick.

Each portion (½ of the recipe) provides: 6 PR, 1 VEG

Sauerbraten Beef Roll

Serves 4

2 pounds flank (or top round) steak, thin-cut for rolling
1½ tablespoons prepared mustard
8 tablespoons plain low-fat yogurt

1½ tablespoons dried onions
3 tablespoons dried mushrooms
1½ teaspoons mixed poultry herbs
1¼ cups dry red wine or tomato juice

Spread beef on one side with mustard. Stir together remaining ingredients, except wine (or juice); spread over steak. Roll steak tightly; cover and refrigerate 24 to 48 hours. Pour on wine (or juice). Cover and roast in a preheated 350-degree oven, 1 hour.

Uncover and roast until meat is very tender, 30 to 45 minutes more. Baste occasionally and add more wine, juice or a little water, if needed. Slice thin to serve.

Each portion (¼ of the recipe) provides: 6 PR

Italian Lemon Steak

Serves 4

2 pounds (about) thick boneless top round steak
1 onion, chopped
2 cloves garlic, minced
½ cup each fresh lemon juice and water

2 tablespoons each fresh (or 2 teaspoons each dried) basil, oregano, and thyme
Salt, coarse pepper, to taste

Trim meat of all fat. Combine remaining ingredients, except salt and pepper; use as a marinade for the steak. Follow the preceding directions. Season to taste at serving time.

Each portion (¼ of the recipe) provides: 6 PR

(continued)

ITALIAN LEMON STEAK, CONTINUED

VARIATION

Hawaiian Round Steak

Follow the preceding directions, substituting Hawaiian Marinade (see page 200) for all ingredients except meat.

Each portion (¼ of the recipe) provides: 6 PR

Baked Steak Diablo   Serves 6

3 pounds top round steak, at least 2 inches thick	2 teaspoons plain (or garlic-seasoned) meat tenderizer
2 tablespoons dark spicy prepared mustard	Coarse black pepper

Trim any fringe fat from steak. Spread meat liberally on both sides with mustard and sprinkle with tenderizer and pepper. Puncture all over with the tines of a fork. Leave at room temperature 30 minutes.

Arrange steak on a rack in a baking pan. Put the pan in a cold oven and set the temperature to 275 degrees. Bake uncovered 2 hours, or until tender. Baste occasionally with pan juices.

Each portion (⅙ of the recipe) provides: 6 PR

Stir-Fried Steak and Asparagus   Serves 2

1 pound fat-trimmed top round steak	1 clove garlic, minced
¾ cup beef broth (or water)	1 teaspoon ground ginger
1 pound fresh asparagus, diagonally sliced into 1-inch pieces	1 tablespoon each cornstarch, soy sauce, and dry sherry or other white wine

Coat a large nonstick skillet or electric frypan with cooking spray. Add steak; brown on both sides over moderate heat. Transfer steak to a cutting board.

Combine broth, asparagus, garlic, and ginger in the skillet. Simmer uncovered, just until asparagus is tender-crunchy, 3 to 5 minutes depending on thickness.

Meanwhile, slice the steak very thin (it will still be raw inside). Blend cornstarch with soy sauce and wine to make a paste; stir into skillet, until sauce simmers and thickens. Stir in the steak slices and heat through to desired doneness.

Each portion (½ of the recipe) provides: 6 PR, 2 VEG

Carne Asada-Style Flank Steak   Serves 2

½ cup lime juice	¼ teaspoon garlic powder
1 to 3 teaspoons chili powder	1 pound (about) beef flank steak
1 teaspoon dried oregano	

Combine juice, chili, oregano, and garlic; pour over steak. Refrigerate 1 to 2 days.

Remove steak from marinade. Broil or barbecue 2 to 4 inches from heat source, about 5 minutes each side, depending on thickness and desired degree of cooking. Slice very thin against the grain to serve.

VARIATIONS

Lemon Steak Italiano

Substitute lemon juice for lime juice. Omit chili powder.

East Indian Steak

Use lime or lemon juice. Substitute curry powder for chili powder. Use mint leaves in place of oregano.

Each portion (½ of the recipe) provides: 6 PR

Steak Siciliano   Serves 4

2 onions, diced
1 sweet red pepper, diced
1 or 2 cloves garlic,
   minced
16-ounce can crushed
   tomatoes

8-ounce can plain tomato
   sauce
2 pounds (about) flank
   steak

Spray a large nonstick skillet generously with cooking spray; heat. Cook onions, red pepper, and garlic 2 to 3 minutes, until vegetables are soft. Add tomatoes and tomato sauce; mix well. Cook 45 minutes, or until sauce thickens.

Brush steak lightly with some of the sauce. Broil or barbecue 4 inches from heat source, 5 minutes. Turn meat and brush again with sauce. Broil 4 to 5 minutes longer, depending on thickness of steak and desired degree of doneness. Slice diagonally in thin slices; serve with remaining sauce.

Each portion (¼ of the recipe) provides: 6 PR, 2 VEG

Hearty London Broil   Serves 4

2 tablespoons each dry red
   wine, lemon juice,
   prepared mustard, and
   Worcestershire sauce

2 pounds (about) beef flank
   steak

Combine wine, juice, mustard, and Worcestershire; spread over the steak. Place steak in a plastic bag; close bag and set it in a bowl. Marinate steak 1 hour at room temperature or refrigerate overnight.

Broil or barbecue steak 2 inches from heat source, 4 to 5 minutes each side (or to desired doneness). Slice thin against the grain to serve.

VARIATIONS

Far Eastern Marinated Flank Steak

Replace red wine with sherry or other white wine. Replace Worcestershire with soy sauce. Add 1 clove minced garlic and 1 teaspoon ground ginger to the marinade.

Steak Iberia

Replace red wine with dry sherry or other white wine, and lemon juice with tomato juice.

Mideastern Steak

Replace wine with mixed-vegetable juice. Add grated peel of 1 lemon. Omit mustard. Add 2 tablespoons fresh basil leaves (or 2 teaspoons dried basil) and 1 teaspoon ground cinnamon.

Each portion (¼ of the recipe) provides: 6 PR

Barbecued London Broil   Serves 6

3 pounds (about) thick
   boneless top round
   steak
½ cup each white wine,
   water
3 tablespoons each lemon
   juice, soy, and
   Worcestershire sauce

1 tablespoon each
   prepared mustard and
   meat tenderizer
Optional: 2 cloves minced
   garlic, coarse black
   pepper

Trim meat of all fat. Put meat in a plastic bag and place bag in a shallow bowl (to catch any drippings). Combine the rest of the ingredients into a marinade and add mixture

(continued)

to bag. Refrigerate 24 hours. Remove meat from the marinade, and broil or barbecue 4 inches from heat source until medium rare inside.

To serve, remove the meat to a cutting board and slice very thin against the grain.

Each portion (⅙ of the recipe) provides: 6 PR

Meat Tacos   Serves 4

Spicy but not hot, unless you top it with a hot sauce.

1 small onion, minced	½ cup plain or spicy tomato
1 clove garlic, minced	juice (or light beer)
2 tablespoons water	1 teaspoon cumin seeds
3 cups chopped cooked	Pinch of dried oregano
lean beef (or chicken	4 corn tortillas
or turkey)	

Coat a large nonstick skillet or electric frying pan with cooking spray. Add onion, garlic, and water. Cook and stir over high heat until water evaporates and onion begins to brown. Stir in meat, juice, cumin, and oregano. Simmer uncovered, stirring often, until most liquid evaporates, about 10 minutes.

Meanwhile, gently heat tortillas, a few at a time, on a nonstick skillet over moderate heat, about 20 seconds per side. Spoon meat mixture into soft tortillas and roll. Serve with Zesty Salsa (see page 188) and shredded lettuce, if desired.

Each portion (1 filled taco) provides: 5 PR, 1 ST

Spicy Cajun Kebobs

Serves 4

2 pounds round steak
  Cajun Marinade (see
    page 199)
4 onions, quartered

4 bell peppers (use red,
  green, and yellow bell
  peppers for best effect)

Trim meat of all fat. Cut meat into 1½-inch cubes and combine with Cajun Marinade. Refrigerate 6 to 8 hours.

At dinnertime, peel and quarter onions; separate into "leaves." Cut peppers into squares; discard seeds, tops, and membranes. Thread the cubes of meat on skewers, alternating with pieces of onion and pepper. Brush vegetables with reserved marinade. Broil or barbecue 3 to 4 inches from heat source 12 to 14 minutes, turning once.

Each portion (¼ of the recipe) provides: 6 PR, 1 VEG

Spicy Sweet and Sour Meatballs

Serves 2

1 pound lean ground beef
  (round)
2 tablespoons minced
  onions
2 tablespoons minced
  parsley
1 tablespoon prepared,
  spicy mustard
1 clove of garlic, minced

8 ounces plain tomato
  sauce
¾ cup water
2 tablespoons light soy
  sauce
2 tablespoons lemon juice
3 packets low-calorie
  sweetener

Mix meat, onion, parsley, mustard, and garlic thoroughly. Shape into 8 meatballs. Brown in a nonstick skillet with no added fat. Turn to brown evenly. Drain and discard fat. Add remaining ingredients, except for sweetener.

Cover and simmer 20 to 25 minutes. Uncover and simmer until sauce is thick. Remove from heat. Stir in sweetener.

Each portion (½ of the recipe) provides: 6 PR

Spinach Meat Loaf   Serves 2

This meat loaf is good as a hot meal or as a cold lunch. For example, you can make a small pita bread sandwich of meat loaf with fresh, sliced tomato.

1 pound lean ground
    round beef or veal (or
    ½ pound beef and ½
    pound veal)
10-ounce package of
    cooked, drained,
    chopped spinach

1 large egg
2 tablespoons minced
    onion
Salt and pepper to taste

Combine all ingredients and mold in a loaf pan. Turn meat loaf out of loaf pan into a nonstick baking pan. Bake at 350 degrees for 45 minutes. Allow to rest a few minutes before slicing.

Each portion (½ of the recipe) provides: 6 PR, 1 VEG

Veal Marengo   Serves 4

2 pounds boneless lean
    veal shoulder,
    trimmed of fat and cut
    into 1-inch cubes
Salt and pepper to taste
½ cup broth or bouillon
½ cup chopped onion

1 clove garlic, minced
1 medium-sized green
    bell pepper, seeded
    and cut into strips
16-ounce can tomatoes, cut
    up
¼ cup dry wine

Season veal with salt and pepper. Brown in a large, sprayed, heavy saucepan over medium high heat. Remove veal and set it aside.

Add broth or bouillon to pan. Add onion and garlic; cook until onion is tender and liquid has almost evaporated. Add bell pepper, tomato, wine, and veal. Cover and simmer for

1 hour, stirring occasionally. Uncover and simmer 15 minutes, or until the veal is tender and sauce has thickened.

Serve hot over toast. If toast is used, one slice will add one serving of starch.

Each portion (¼ of the recipe) provides: 6 PR

Oven Shish Kebob

Serves 4

2 pounds lean leg-of-lamb steak	Optional: few drops liquid smoke (or hickory-seasoned salt) and pepper
¾ cup plain low-fat yogurt	
1 clove garlic, minced	
½ teaspoon each dried mint and marjoram (or oregano)	2 onions
	2 bell peppers, 1 red, 1 green

Cut lamb into 1½-inch cubes; discard fat and center bone. Combine with yogurt, garlic, herbs, and seasoning. Refrigerate all day or overnight.

Peel and quarter onions, separate into leaves. Cut off tops of the peppers; remove membranes and seeds. Cut peppers into 1½-inch squares. Alternate the meat cubes on skewers with onion leaves and pepper squares. Brush skewers lightly with any remaining marinade.

Suspend the skewers over the edges of a shallow baking pan. Put the pan in a preheated, very hot, 450-degree oven for 30 to 40 minutes.

Each portion (¼ of the recipe) provides: 6 PR, 1 VEG

Lamb Rogan Josh

Serves 4

You think the British prefer food bland and boring? Not so! They love hot and spicy Indian curries with the same passion Americans have for Mexican food. Curried lamb Rogan Josh

(continued)

LAMB ROGAN JOSH, CONTINUED

*is so popular that Britons can buy it frozen—like American
frozen pizza or chili.*

1¼ pounds cooked lamb, cut in cubes	1 tablespoon cornstarch
2 cups canned-in-puree tomatoes	1 teaspoon each (or more, to taste) cumin and fennel seeds, and curry powder
4 tablespoons raisins	
Half of a small onion, minced	¼ teaspoon each ground cinnamon, ginger, and allspice
1 clove garlic, minced	

Combine all ingredients in a saucepan and stir well. Cover,
simmer 10 minutes. Serve with rice (½ cup rice provides 1
ST).

Each portion (¼ of the recipe) provides: 5 PR, ¼ FR

Roast Leg of Lamb

Leg of lamb
Salt and pepper to taste
Seasonings of your choice
   (some suggestions:
   Middle Eastern: lemon
   juice, mint, garlic,
cinnamon, and nutmeg;
French: white wine,
garlic, tarragon, onion;
Italian: red wine, garlic,
oregano, basil, onion)

Preheat oven to 325 degrees. Sprinkle lamb with salt, pepper and other seasonings. Place roast fat side up on a rack
in an open roasting pan. Insert a meat thermometer in the
meatiest part, not touching bone.

Roast uncovered with no fat added until meat reaches
the desired degree of doneness: rare: 140 to 150 degrees;
medium: 155–165 degrees; well done: 175 degrees.

Remove roast from the oven and let it rest for 10 to 15 minutes before serving.

Pork Plum Kebobs

Serves 2

1 pound fresh ham steak (pork leg)
2 tablespoons each vinegar and soy sauce
1 tablespoon plum preserves

Optional: dash of 5-spice powder or pumpkin pie spice
4 fresh purple plums
1 onion

Slice meat into 1½-inch chunks; combine with vinegar, soy sauce, preserves, and spice (if you are using it). Cut unpeeled plums in half and remove the pits. Cut each half into 4 thick slices. Peel and quarter the onion and separate into leaves. Alternate the meat cubes with onion and plum slices on skewers.

Broil or barbecue 3 inches from heat source about 20 to 25 minutes, turning occasionally and brushing with the marinade, until meat is cooked through.

Each portion (½ of the recipe) provides: 6 PR, 1 FR

Ham Steak Hawaiian

Serves 2

1 pound ready-to-eat ham slice

1 cup juice-packed crushed pineapple
Pinch of ground clove

Trim fringe fat from ham; brown in skillet over medium heat. Turn and brown other side. Remove to a platter.

Add pineapple and clove to the skillet. Cook and stir over high heat until heated through. Pour pineapple sauce over ham steak to serve.

Each portion (½ of the recipe) provides: 6 PR, ½ FR

Chicken and Peppers   Serves 4

2 pounds chicken thighs
    (skin removed)
12 ounces tomato juice
4 tablespoons light Italian
    salad dressing

2 cups each sliced onion
    and sliced Italian
    frying peppers

Put chicken in a nonstick skillet over moderate heat. Cook slowly, turning frequently. Discard any melted fat from skillet.

Add tomato juice and dressing. Cover and simmer 20 minutes. Uncover; add onions and peppers. Cook uncovered, about 25 minutes, stirring frequently, until chicken is tender and sauce is reduced.

Each portion (¼ of the recipe) provides: 5 PR, 2 VEG

Chicken Mushroom Supreme   Serves 4

4 chicken cutlets
    (boneless, skinless
    breast fillets)

16 ounces sliced
    mushrooms (fresh or
    canned)
1 cup dry sherry (or
    vermouth)

Coat a large nonstick skillet with cooking spray and add the chicken cutlets in a single layer. Cook over moderate heat 4 minutes. Transfer to a heated platter.

Put the mushrooms and wine in the skillet and turn the heat high. Cook and stir until most of the wine has evaporated. Spoon the mushrooms over the chicken and serve immediately.

Each portion (¼ of the recipe) provides: 6 PR, 1 VEG

Breast of Chicken Cacciatore   Serves 4

6 ounces tomato juice
5 tablespoons dry white
    wine
1 large vine-ripe tomato,
    peeled and cubed
1 bell pepper, seeded and
    diced
1 small onion, thinly sliced

1 tablespoon fresh basil
    and/or oregano (or 1
    teaspoon dried Italian
    herbs)
Salt (or garlic salt),
    pepper, to taste
4 broiled chicken breasts
    (skin removed)

Combine all ingredients, except chicken, in a saucepan.
Cover and simmer 15 minutes.

Meanwhile, on a cutting board, slice the chicken into
cubes and discard the bones. Uncover pan and stir in the
chicken. Simmer uncovered, until sauce is thick.

Each portion (¼ of the recipe) provides: 6 PR, ½ VEG

Chicken Cutlets with Mushrooms and Onions   Serves 2

2 skinless, boneless chicken
    breasts (about 1 pound)
1 large sweet onion, halved
    and sliced

2 cups sliced fresh
    mushrooms
Pinch of grated nutmeg
Salt (or seasoned salt)
    and coarse pepper

Coat a large nonstick skillet or electric frying pan liberally
with cooking spray. Add the chicken and onion slices in a
shallow layer. Brown the chicken and onions with no fat
added, over moderate heat for 3 to 4 minutes. Turn the
chicken and stir in the mushroom slices. Cover the skillet
and cook over low heat 4 to 5 minutes more, just until
chicken is cooked through and onions and mushrooms are
tender-crunchy. Season to taste and serve immediately; pile
the onions and mushrooms on top of the chicken cutlets.

Each portion (½ of the recipe) provides: 6 PR, ½ VEG

Drumsticks Diablo   Serves 3

6 frying chicken drumsticks   2 tablespoons Dijon-style
3 tablespoons plain low-fat   mustard
   yogurt   Salt (or seasoned salt),
                       pepper, to taste

Remove the skin from the drumsticks. Put drumsticks in a
plastic bag with remaining ingredients. Shake until well
coated. Or combine coating ingredients and slather over
drumsticks. Arrange on a rack in a roasting pan. Bake uncovered in a preheated 400-degree oven 35 to 40 minutes.

Each portion (⅓ of the recipe) provides: 6 PR

Chicken Florentine   Serves 2

1 10-ounce package frozen,   2 cups cooked, chopped
   chopped spinach,   chicken or turkey
   thawed   2 tablespoons grated
1 teaspoon lemon juice   Parmesan cheese
   Salt and pepper to taste

Place the thawed spinach in a 1-quart casserole that has
been coated with cooking spray. Sprinkle lemon juice, salt,
and pepper over spinach. Cover with chicken (or turkey).
Sprinkle with Parmesan cheese. Bake in 350-degree oven
about 20 minutes or until heated through and the spinach
is cooked.

Each portion (½ of the recipe) provides: 6 PR, 1 VEG

Chicken with Pineapple Garnish   Serves 2

½ cup soy sauce   2 large skinned chicken
1 small clove garlic,   breasts, split
   minced   3 pineapple rings
                     Parsley for garnish

Mix soy sauce and garlic; marinate chicken breasts for 2 hours in soy sauce mixture.

Place chicken on foil-lined pan coated with cooking spray. Spoon marinade over the chicken and bake, covered, for 1 hour at 350 degrees; then uncover and continue baking for 10 to 15 minutes more.

Broil pineapple. Use it, along with the parsley, to garnish.

Each portion (½ of the recipe) provides: 6 PR, 1 FR

Citrus Chicken Spinach Salad   Serves 2

10-ounce package raw
   spinach
2 cups diced cooked
   chicken
2 oranges, peeled, seeded,
   and cubed
1 red onion, halved and
   thinly sliced

Dressing:
3 tablespoons orange juice
2 tablespoons each lemon
   juice and light soy
   sauce
1 teaspoon each prepared
   hot mustard, ground
   ginger

Wash spinach in cold water and tear into bite-size pieces. Divide between 2 salad bowls. Arrange remaining salad ingredients on top. Combine dressing ingredients in a covered jar, shake well and pour over salads.

Each portion (½ of the recipe) provides: 5 PR, 1 FR, 2 VEG

Tahitian Turkey

1 cup chicken bouillon
1½ teaspoons ground
   ginger
8 to 10 pound turkey, cut
   into parts, or 8 to 10
   pound turkey breast

12 ounce can of orange
   juice
½ cup light soy sauce

Combine chicken bouillon and ginger; mix well. Remove skin from turkey pieces. Coat roasting pan with cooking

(continued)

spray, then place turkey in it and brush with some of the
bouillon mixture.

Bake at 375 degrees, covered, for 1¼ hours. Turn in pan.
Combine orange juice, soy sauce, and remaining bouillon
mixture; pour over the turkey. Continue baking until turkey
is done, basting often. Slice into desired portions.

Six ounces of cooked turkey provides: 6 PR

Middle Eastern Baked Sea Steaks   Serves 4

1½ pounds swordfish,   6 tablespoons plain low-
    salmon, or other fish   fat yogurt
    steaks   Optional: minced fresh
10 or 12 bay leaves   parsley and chives
4 tablespoons lemon juice

Arrange fish steaks on top of bay leaves in a single layer.
Sprinkle with lemon juice. Bake in a preheated, very hot,
450-degree oven, 15 to 20 minutes, only until fish flakes
(don't overcook). Put fish steaks on a platter.

Discard bay leaves. Fork-blend yogurt with pan drippings. Spoon yogurt mixture over fish; sprinkle with minced
parsley and chives. Serve immediately.

Each portion (¼ of the recipe) provides: 5 PR

Barbecued Swordfish Steaks   Serves 2

2 swordfish steaks   Garlic salt, pepper
    (about 1 pound)   Mesquite or hickory chips
    Bay leaves   (or liquid smoke
    Juice of 2 limes   seasoning)

If swordfish steaks are frozen, put them in a plastic bag
with bay leaves, lime juice, garlic salt, and pepper. Allow
them to defrost slowly in the refrigerator. For fresh or

thawed swordfish, put the steaks in a bag with seasoning ingredients for 30 minutes at room temperature.

To barbecue: If you are using wood chips for flavoring smoke, soak them in hot water 20 minutes, then put them on the hot coals. Arrange fish steaks 5 inches from heat source, and slow cook them in the smoke about 10 to 12 minutes per side. Or arrange the fish steaks in a hinged revolving rotisserie basket and barbecue them in the revolving grill about 20 minutes, just until fish starts to flake. Be very careful not to overcook the fish because it will dry out.

To broil indoors, spray or sprinkle fish with smoke seasoning just before broiling 3 inches from heat source, about 5 minutes per side. For best results, swordfish steaks should be 1 inch thick. Shorten cooking time for thinner fish. Remove bay leaves before serving.

Each portion (½ of the recipe) provides: 6 PR

Brook Trout with Leek and Fennel

From Adrian's Café in Philadelphia. Use this method with any small whole fish.

Fresh brook trout	Dry white wine
Fresh leeks and fennel	Salt and pepper
Thin lemon slices	

For each fish: Cut a circle of parchment paper (available in culinary specialty stores, or use aluminum foil) about 2 inches larger than the fish. Thinly slice fresh leek and fennel (bulb part only); use about 1 ounce of each per fish. Arrange the fish on top of the parchment and add slices of leek, fennel, and lemon. Sprinkle with 1 tablespoon white wine; salt and pepper to taste.

Fold the paper over the fish and then pleat the edges.

(continued)

BROOK TROUT WITH LEEK AND FENNEL, CONTINUED

Arrange fish packets in a single layer in a baking dish. Bake 8 minutes at 350 degrees.

Each trout (average size) provides: 6 PR

Saucy Catfish Fillets   Serves 4

1¼ pounds fresh catfish
    fillets (or other fish
    fillets)
3 tablespoons low-fat
    mayonnaise

1 tablespoon lemon juice
Seasoned salt, pepper,
    to taste

Cut catfish fillets into serving pieces; combine in a plastic bag with mayonnaise and lemon juice. Close bag tightly and shake until fillets are evenly coated.

Spray a shallow nonstick baking pan with cooking spray. Arrange catfish in a single layer. Sprinkle lightly with seasoned salt and pepper. Bake uncovered in a preheated, very hot 450-degree oven 10 to 12 minutes, depending on thickness of fillets. Fish is done when it just begins to flake; don't overcook.

Each portion (¼ of the recipe) provides: 5 PR

Sour Creamy Flounder Fillets   Serves 2

1¼ pounds fresh thawed
    flounder (or other
    fish fillets)
1 small onion, thinly
    sliced
½ cup dry white wine,
    divided

6 tablespoons plain low-
    fat yogurt
Seasoned salt and
    pepper to taste
2 tablespoons fresh dill
    (or parsley), minced
Optional: paprika

Spray a nonstick baking dish with cooking spray. Cut fish fillets into 4 equal servings. Arrange the fillets over several onion slices. Pour on half the wine. Bake uncovered, in a preheated 450-degree oven 12 to 14 minutes, depending on thickness of the fillets. Add more wine if needed. Transfer fish to serving dish.

Add remaining wine and yogurt to baking dish and blend with fork. Spoon over fish. Sprinkle with salt, pepper, dill, and paprika before serving.

Each portion (½ of the recipe) provides: 6 PR

Italian-Style Fish Fillets   Serves 2

1 small onion, minced
1¼ pounds fish fillets (sole, flounder, or halibut), fresh or thawed
4 tablespoons low-fat calorie-reduced Italian-style salad dressing

2 tablespoons chopped fresh parsley
¼ cup grated Parmesan (or Romano) cheese

Sprinkle onion in an ovenproof dish. Top with fillets in a single layer. Spread with dressing. Sprinkle with parsley and cheese. Cover and bake in a preheated 450-degree oven for 10 minutes. Uncover and bake 4 to 6 minutes more, until browned.

Each portion (½ of the recipe) provides: 5 PR

Halibut in Wine   Serves 6

3 pounds halibut or other fish fillets

1 cup white wine
Salt, pepper, paprika

Arrange fish fillets in an oven-to-table casserole dish. Add the wine. Sprinkle with salt and pepper to taste. Bake at 350 degrees, 10 minutes, until fish whitens. Sprinkle with paprika before serving.

Each portion (⅙ of the recipe) provides: 6 PR

15 Meal-Size Soups

Beef and Barley Soup

Serves 8

Meaty bones left over from beef roast	4 tablespoons medium pearl barley
20-ounce can Italian tomatoes	4 onions, peeled and quartered
5 cups water	1 carrot, sliced
2 teaspoons salt (or garlic salt)	1 cup chopped bell pepper
1 teaspoon each: fennel seeds, dried oregano (or Italian seasoning)	¼ cup minced fresh (preferably Italian) parsley
	Optional: sprinkle of Parmesan cheese

Combine meaty bones, tomatoes, water and seasonings. Cover and simmer 1½ hours (or 30 minutes in pressure cooker) until meat falls easily from bones.

Refrigerate until cool. Remove and discard hardened fat from surface of soup. Remove meat from bones; discard bones. Reheat soup and meat. Add remaining ingredients, except cheese. Cover and simmer until barley is tender, about 45 minutes. Serve with a scant sprinkle of cheese, if desired.

VARIATION

Turkey and Barley Soup

Substitute meaty bones left over from roast turkey.

Each portion (⅛ of the recipe) provides: 1 PR, 1 VEG, ⅛ ST

Scotch Broth   Serves 6

Meaty bones from roast
  leg of lamb
2 quarts water
2 or 3 bay leaves
Salt to taste
¼ teaspoon pepper

½ cup each sliced onion,
  carrot, celery, and
  turnip
4 tablespoons barley
½ teaspoon dried marjoram

Place meaty lamb bones in a large pot with water, bay
leaves, salt, and pepper. Bring to a boil; skin and discard
any foam from soup. Cover and simmer 1½ hours.

Cool soup; skim and discard any fat from surface. Remove bones and dice the lamb. Discard bones and return
meat to the soup along with remaining ingredients. Cover
and simmer 45 minutes more, stirring occasionally. Remove bay leaves before serving.

Each portion (⅙ of the recipe) provides: 1 PR, ⅙ ST, ½ VEG

Turkey Scotch Broth   Serves 8

Meaty bones left over
  from roast turkey
2 quarts water
Optional: 2 teaspoons salt
4 tablespoons medium
  pearl barley
4 carrots, sliced

4 ribs celery with leaves,
  cut in 1¼ inch lengths
2 onions, peeled and
  quartered
¼ cup minced fresh parsley

Combine turkey bones in a stock pot with water and salt.
Cover; simmer 1½ hours (or 30 minutes in a pressure
cooker) until meat falls easily from bones.

Refrigerate. When cool, remove and discard hardened
fat from surface of soup. Remove meat from bones; reserve
meat and discard bones. Reheat soup and meat. Add barley

(continued)

and vegetables. Cover and simmer until barley is tender,
about 45 minutes.

Each portion (⅛ of the recipe) provides: 1 PR, ⅛ ST. ½ VEG

Basic Chicken Broth
*Basic chicken broth can be used in soups or as cooking liquid
for vegetables. (They'll taste great without adding any butter
or margarine.) Use the meat for salads, sandwiches, and other
recipes.*

1 whole (or cut-up) frying chicken	Salt, pepper, seasonings, to taste
Water, onion, and celery	Optional: bay leaf, pinch of thyme

You can use whole chicken (which is cheaper) or cut-up
parts (all white meat or dark, your preference). If you use
whole chicken, it is not necessary to disjoint it, but do add
the neck and giblets to the pot to flavor the broth. It is not
necessary to remove the skin.

Put the chicken in a heavy covered pot and add 1 cup of
water for each pound of chicken. Add a peeled onion and a
rib of cut-up celery or some celery leaves. Add 1 teaspoon
salt per pound (or to taste) and other seasonings to taste.

Cover pot tightly and simmer over low heat 45 minutes
to 1 hour, until chicken is tender. Remove pot from heat
and leave chicken in the broth until cool enough to handle.
When chicken is cool, remove and discard skin, bones, and
bay leaf, if you are using it. Wrap and refrigerate meat for
use in other recipes.

Strain broth and refrigerate. When cool, skim and discard the fat that forms on the surface. Refrigerate broth or,
for longer storage, freeze.

Speedy Chicken Noodle Vegetable Soup   Serves 4

4 cups fat-skimmed
    chicken broth, fresh or
    canned
1 cup fine egg noodles
2 carrots, unpared

1 small onion
1 rib celery
3 tablespoons minced fresh
    parsley

Heat broth to boiling; add noodles a few at a time. Put vegetables through coarse shredding disk, then add them to the boiling soup. Simmer 5 more minutes.

Each portion (¼ of the recipe) provides: 1 ST, ½ VEG

Chicken Soup Primavera   Serves 2

3 cups chicken broth, fat
    skimmed
2 large ribs celery, thinly
    sliced
½ cup chopped sweet
    onion
10-ounce package frozen
    Italian-style (or
    Oriental) mixed
    vegetables

1 cup sliced mushrooms
3 tablespoons minced
    parsley
Optional: a few fresh sage
    (or thyme) leaves,
    minced
6 ounces cooked chicken
    breast, diced

Heat broth to boiling. Add celery and onion. Simmer 5 minutes. Add remaining ingredients, except chicken. Simmer just until vegetables are crispy-crunchy, about 6 to 7 minutes more. Stir in cooked chicken and heat through.

Each portion (½ of the recipe) provides: 3 PR, 2 VEG

Spanish Salad Soup   Serves 6

1 cucumber, peeled and chopped
1 small onion, minced
½ bell pepper, diced
2 cups plain (or spicy) tomato juice
1 cup mixed-vegetable juice

3 tablespoons olive liquid (from jar of olives)
2 tablespoons each lemon juice and minced parsley (or cilantro)
Optional: paprika, hot pepper, minced garlic (to taste)

Combine ingredients and chill thoroughly before serving.

Each portion (⅙ of the recipe) provides: 1 VEG

Minestrone Medley   Serves 8

2 cups dried lentils
6 cups fresh cold water
6-ounce can tomato paste
3 ribs celery, minced
1 cup each coarsely chopped cabbage and sliced mushrooms
1 onion, chopped

1 teaspoon each garlic salt and Italian herbs (or ½ teaspoon each dried oregano and basil)
Pepper to taste
Pinch of hot pepper flakes
8 tablespoons grated Parmesan cheese

Soak lentils overnight in water; drain and discard water. Combine lentils with 6 cups fresh cold water. Heat to boiling. Stir in remaining ingredients, except cheese. Cover and simmer 45 minutes. Serve sprinkled with Parmesan.

Each portion (⅛ of the recipe) provides: ½ PR, 1 ST

Tuna Skillet Gumbo   Serves 4

16 ounces stewed tomatoes
10 ounces frozen okra,
   thawed
1 cup each sliced onion,
   diced (red and green)
   bell pepper and water
6-ounce can clam-tomato
   (or mixed-vegetable)
   juice

2 cloves garlic, minced
¼ teaspoon dried thyme
1 cup uncooked long
   grain rice
14 ounces water-packed
   solid white tuna

Combine ingredients, except rice and tuna; heat to boiling.
Lower heat, cover and simmer 5 minutes. Stir in rice and
simmer 15 minutes more; stir occasionally.

Break tuna into large flakes and arrange on top of ingredients, along with liquid from cans. Cover and simmer just
until heated through.

Each portion (¼ of the recipe) provides: 3½ PR, 1 ST, 1 VEG

16 Potatoes, Pasta, and Rice

Range-Top Rice Dressing

Serves 8

1 cup each raw brown rice, chopped onion, chopped celery, fat-skimmed chicken or turkey broth, and boiling water
4-ounce can mushroom stems and pieces, undrained

1 teaspoon poultry seasoning (or ½ teaspoon each dried sage and thyme)
Salt (or garlic salt), pepper, to taste
4 tablespoons chopped fresh parsley

Combine all ingredients except parsley. Cover and simmer 50 to 60 minutes in a nonstick pan. Fluff with a fork and stir in parsley just before serving. Serve with roast chicken or turkey.

Each portion (⅛ of the recipe, or ½ cup dressing) provides: 1 ST

Rice Primavera Pronto

Serves 6

10-ounce can fat-skimmed undiluted chicken broth
½ cup each shredded raw carrots, zucchini, and yellow squash

1 cup instant rice
3 tablespoons sliced scallion (or onion)

Combine chicken broth and shredded carrots; simmer 1 minute. Remove from heat and stir in remaining ingredients. Keep tightly covered 5 minutes or more. Fluff with a fork before serving.

Each portion (⅙ of the recipe) provides: 1 ST

Rice Jardin   Serves 6

1½ cups boiling water	½ teaspoon dried tarragon
1 cup tomato (or mixed-vegetable) juice	(or rosemary or mixed herbs)
½ cup each sliced onion, sliced celery, and chopped bell pepper	1 cup long-grain uncooked rice
1 tablespoon Worcestershire (or soy) sauce	10-ounce package frozen mixed vegetables

Combine ingredients, except rice and frozen vegetables. Heat to boiling. Stir in rice; reheat to boiling. Arrange block of frozen vegetables on top. Simmer 25 to 30 minutes, until liquid is absorbed and rice is tender. Fluff with a fork to mix in vegetables.

Each portion (⅙ of the recipe) provides: 1 ST

Cottage Stuffed Potatoes   Serves 8

4 large baking potatoes	minced fresh parsley, and
1 cup pot-style low-fat cottage cheese	plain low-fat yogurt
3 tablespoons each chopped chives (or scallions or onions),	Optional: paprika and lemon pepper

Pierce potatoes and bake whole in a preheated 425-degree oven 40 to 60 minutes, or until tender, or in microwave oven according to manufacturer's directions.

(continued)

COTTAGE STUFFED POTATOES, CONTINUED

Remove from oven and when cool enough to handle, slice each potato in half. Gently scoop out most, but not all, of potato; combine with cheese, chives, parsley, and yogurt. Mash or beat together in electric mixer bowl, or process with pulse setting of food processor, until mixture is combined. Spoon into potato shells. Arrange in a single layer on a nonstick shallow baking tray or cookie tin sprayed with cooking spray. Bake uncovered in a preheated 425-degree oven until heated through and tops are golden, about 20 minutes. Sprinkle with paprika and lemon pepper if desired.

Each portion (⅛ of the recipe) provides: 1 ST, ½ PR

Potato Bake Parmesan

Small baking potatoes	Oregano and basil
Thin onion slices	Garlic salt and pepper
Tomato juice	Grated Parmesan cheese

For each potato, make several slits about ¼ inch apart, not cutting all the way through. Slip a small thin slice of onion into each slit. Combine 2 teaspoons tomato juice with a pinch of the herbs, garlic salt, and pepper; spoon mixture over the potato.

Wrap each potato tightly in double-thick or heavy-duty sprayed aluminum foil and cook 1 hour in a covered barbecue, or in the oven. Unwrap each potato packet carefully and sprinkle with 1 tablespoon Parmesan before serving. Cheese will melt.

Each portion (small baking potato) provides: ½ PR, 1 ST

Scalloped Potato Casserole

Serves 4

2 cups thinly sliced
potatoes
½ cup each dried
mushrooms and
thinly sliced onions
1¼ cups fat-skimmed
condensed beef (or
chicken) broth,
undiluted

Pinch of grated nutmeg
and shake of paprika
3 tablespoons finely
chopped parsley

Combine ingredients, except parsley, in a covered baking
dish and bake in a preheated 350-degree oven 45 minutes.
Uncover and bake, basting occasionally, 10 to 15 minutes
longer. Sprinkle with parsley before serving.

Each portion (¼ of the recipe) provides: 1 ST

Veggie Vermicelli

Serves 8

4 cups hot, tender-cooked,
drained thin spaghetti
(vermicelli)
½ cup each shredded raw
carrot, yellow squash,
and zucchini
Small onion, halved and
sliced thin
½ cup each fat-skimmed
chicken broth and
white wine

2 teaspoons fresh (or pinch
dried) basil
Pinch each grated
nutmeg and lemon
peel
Salt (or garlic salt) and
coarse pepper
4 tablespoons grated
Parmesan cheese
2 tablespoons minced
fresh parsley

Cook spaghetti in boiling salted water, then drain. Combine carrot, yellow squash, zucchini, onion, broth, and wine
in the pot the spaghetti was cooked in. Simmer uncovered

(continued)

VEGGIE VERMICELLI, CONTINUED

5 minutes. Stir in remaining ingredients, except cheese and parsley. Heat through. Sprinkle with cheese and parsley.

Each portion (⅛ of the recipe) provides: 1 ST, 1 VEG

Shredded Zucchini with Pasta   Serves 4

2 cups cooked high-protein   4 tablespoons lemon juice
   spaghetti (or linguine)   Salt (or garlic salt),
1 zucchini   pepper, to taste
1 sweet red pepper   Optional: 4 tablespoons
1 onion   grated Parmesan

While spaghetti is cooking in boiling (salted) water according to package directions, prepare the vegetables. Shred the zucchini and red pepper by hand or with the shredding disk of a food processor (or, if you prefer, simply dice them into cubes). Cut the onion in half, then thinly slice into spaghettilike strands.

When spaghetti is cooked, drain, then return to the same pot it was cooked in. Stir in all the other ingredients (except the Parmesan) over very low heat, just until heated through. (Or combine ingredients in a microwave-safe serving bowl and heat through at the lowest setting in the microwave oven just before serving.)

Sprinkle with additional minced fresh herbs (and 1 tablespoon grated Parmesan per serving, if desired) just before serving.

Each portion (¼ of the recipe) provides: 1 ST, ½ VEG

The next seven recipes are meal-size combinations that include poultry, meat, or fish.

Chicken-Macaroni Salad

Serves 1

1 cup cooked cubed white-meat chicken
1 tablespoon lemon juice (or vinegar)
½ cup macaroni twists, cooked and chilled
½ cup diagonally sliced celery
½ cup sliced carrots
1 small red onion, chopped

4 tablespoons chopped fresh parsley
2 tablespoons minced fresh basil leaves
2 tablespoons low-calorie mayonnaise
4 tablespoons plain low-fat yogurt
Salt (or garlic salt), coarse pepper

Marinate chicken chunks in lemon juice while you prepare remaining ingredients. Then, toss together lightly and chill until serving time.

Each portion (1 recipe) provides: 5 PR, 1 ST, 1 VEG, ⅓ ML

Cajun Chicken-Rice Casserole

Serves 2

2 cups cooked diced white-meat chicken (or turkey)
2 cups canned tomatoes, undrained
1 cup cooked brown rice

½ cup each chopped onion, minced celery, diced red (or green) sweet bell pepper, and cubed yellow summer squash
1 clove garlic, minced
¼ teaspoon each dried thyme, red pepper, ground clove, and allspice

Layer ingredients in casserole. Bake uncovered in a preheated 350-degree oven 35 to 40 minutes.

Each portion (½ of the recipe) provides: 5 PR, 1 ST, 2 VEG

**One-Pan Chicken and Noodles
with Wine and Mushrooms**   Serves 2

*Ruffled-edge noodles don't need precooking in water. They
cook right in the sauce—the ruffled edges keep them from
sticking together.*

12 ounces chicken (or turkey) thigh cutlets (boneless, skinless dark meat)	6 ounces tomato (or mixed-vegetable) juice
1 cup tiny peeled onions, fresh or frozen	1 cup boiling water
	1 cup dry red wine
4-ounce can mushroom stems and pieces	2 ounces uncooked ruffled-edge curly noodles
1 clove garlic, minced (or pinch of garlic flakes)	2 cups sliced carrots, fresh or thawed
1 or 2 bay leaves	1 to 2 tablespoons minced fresh parsley
½ teaspoon poultry seasoning or ¼ teaspoon each thyme and sage	

Cut the poultry into 1-inch bite-size cubes. Coat a large
nonstick pot with cooking spray; add the cubes; brown over
moderate heat with no fat added.

Stir in the onions, undrained mushrooms, garlic, bay
leaves, and poultry seasoning or thyme and sage. Add tomato juice and water. Cover and simmer 20 to 25 minutes.
Uncover; pour on wine. Place noodles on top. Arrange carrots on top of noodles and sprinkle with parsley. Cover
tightly and simmer 12 to 15 minutes more.

To serve, arrange carrots on a platter or individual plates.
Then stir noodles into the chicken-mushroom-wine mixture, place next to carrots. Remove bay leaves.

Each portion (½ of the recipe) provides: 5 PR, 1 ST, 2 VEC

Turkey Manicotti

Serves 6

1 pound ground raw
  turkey
1 egg (or equivalent
  substitute)
  Garlic salt and pepper to
  taste
1 teaspoon pizza herbs,
  divided
6 uncooked manicotti

16-ounce can tomatoes,
  broken up, undrained
4-ounce can mushrooms,
  undrained
½ cup white wine
3 tablespoons minced
  onion
1 clove garlic, minced

Mix turkey, egg, garlic salt and pepper, and ½ teaspoon
herbs. Stuff mixture into manicotti shells. Place in a single
layer in a nonstick baking pan.

Combine remaining ingredients and add remaining ½
teaspoon herbs. Pour over manicotti. Cover with foil; bake
2 hours at 300 degrees.

Each portion (⅙ of the recipe) provides: 2 PR, 1 ST, 1 VEG

One-Pan Beefburger Noodle Stroganoff

Serves 4

12 ounces fat-trimmed
  ground beef round
2 cups tomato juice
10-ounce can condensed
  beef broth, fat-
  skimmed
4-ounce can mushrooms,
  undrained
1 cup thinly sliced onion
1 teaspoon prepared
  mustard

Dash of Worcestershire
  sauce
Salt (or garlic salt),
  pepper to taste
6 ounces uncooked ruffle-
  edged noodles
½ cup plain low-fat yogurt
Optional: 4 tablespoons
  minced fresh parsley

Spray a nonstick skillet with cooking spray. Brown beef,
breaking into chunks and turning to brown evenly. Drain
and discard any fat from skillet.

(continued)

ONE-PAN BEEFBURGER NOODLE STROGANOFF, CONTINUED

Add tomato juice, broth, mushrooms, onion and seasonings. Heat to boiling. Add noodles, a few at a time. Cover, reduce heat, and simmer until most of the liquid evaporates.

Top each serving with a dollop of yogurt and a sprinkle of parsley.

Each portion (¼ of the recipe) provides: 2½ PR, 1 ST

Linguine with Seafood Sauce   Serves 4

1 pound firm-fleshed fish fillets (monkfish, for example)	4 ounces dry white wine Lemon pepper
6 ounces uncooked linguine	4 ounces plain low-fat yogurt
1 cup sliced fresh mushrooms	4 tablespoons minced fresh dill (or parsley)
1 small onion, sliced	16 tiny cherry tomatoes
	1 cup cubed raw zucchini

Cut fillets into bite-size cubes; set aside. Cook linguine in boiling water (salted, if desired).

Meanwhile, spray a nonstick frying pan with cooking spray. Brown the mushrooms with no fat added. Stir in the onion, wine, and pepper. Cover and simmer over low heat 3 to 4 minutes. Add the fish cubes. Simmer 2 minutes. Remove from the heat and set aside.

Drain linguine; return it to the pan it was cooked in. Stir in yogurt, fish mixture, dill, tomatoes and zucchini. Mix lightly and serve immediately.

Each portion (¼ of the recipe) provides: 2 PR, 1 ST, 1 VEG

Southern Fish and Potato Stew   Serves 4

½ cup cubed lean ham (or Canadian-style bacon)	1 cup boiling water
1 cup chopped onion	2 tablespoons each lemon juice and Worcestershire sauce
28 ounces canned tomatoes	½ teaspoon dried thyme
2 cups diced raw potatoes	Dash of Tabasco
	1½ pounds firm fish fillets

Spray a nonstick pan with cooking spray; brown ham with no fat added. Add onion; cook until tender. Add remaining ingredients, except fish. Cover and simmer for 30 minutes.

Cut fish into 1-inch pieces. Add to pan; cover and simmer just until fish turns opaque, 4 to 6 minutes longer, depending on the kind of fish.

Each portion (¼ of the recipe) provides: 5 PR, 1 ST

17 Vegetables

Fresh, frozen or canned—steamed, simmered, or stir-fried—solo or sauced—hot or cold—green beans are a versatile addition to any low-calorie meal.

Green Beans with Bacon
Serves 4

4 ounces Canadian bacon, diced
1 pound fresh green beans, trimmed, sliced diagonally

½ small onion, thinly sliced
¼ cup water
Salt, freshly ground pepper

Spray a nonstick saucepan lightly with cooking spray. Cook bacon over moderate heat, stirring until lightly browned. Remove from pan; set aside.

Combine beans, onion, and water in the saucepan. Cover; cook until beans are tender-crisp, about 12 minutes. Drain and season to taste. Lightly stir in bacon.

Each portion (¼ of the recipe) provides: 1 PR, 1 VEG

Greek-Style Green Beans
Serves 8

16-ounce can tomatoes
½ cup water
2 onions, finely chopped
3 tablespoons chopped fresh parsley
1 clove garlic, minced
1 tablespoon chopped fresh (or 1 teaspoon dried) mint

2 teaspoons oregano or Italian seasoning
Salt, freshly ground pepper, to taste
1½ pounds fresh (or 20 ounces frozen) green beans

Break up tomatoes with a fork. Combine undrained tomatoes with remaining ingredients, except green beans, in a saucepan. Cover; simmer 10 minutes, stirring frequently.

Meanwhile, wash, tip, and cut up fresh beans (or allow frozen beans to defrost). Add to pot and simmer uncovered, stirring frequently, until beans are tender and sauce is thick.

Each portion (⅛ of the recipe) provides: 1 VEG

Marinated Green Bean Medley   Serves 4

16-ounce package green
    beans, thawed
 1 small onion, chopped
 1 red bell pepper, diced
 4 black (or green) olives,
    sliced
 6 tablespoons olive liquid
    (from olive container)

3 tablespoons vinegar
   Garlic salt, black
     pepper, cayenne
     pepper, oregano (or
     Italian seasoning), to
     taste

Combine ingredients in a glass bowl; season to taste. Cover and chill several hours in refrigerator before serving.

Each portion (¼ of the recipe) provides: 1 VEG

Minty Carrots   Serves 2

10-ounces frozen carrots,
    thawed
 5 or 6 mint leaves, fresh or
    dried

2 tablespoons fruit juice
   (apple, orange, etc.)
   Salt, coarse pepper, to
    taste

Combine ingredients in heavy-duty or double-thick sprayed foil packet and cook on the grill 20 to 25 minutes.

Each portion (½ of the recipe) provides: 1 VEG

Bayou Cauliflower   Serves 5

16-ounce can sliced stewed   1 clove garlic, minced
    tomatoes   ¼ teaspoon each dried
½ cup each, chopped, bell   thyme and marjoram,
    pepper, onion, and   ground clove, allspice,
    celery   and cayenne pepper
3 tablespoons minced   20-ounce bag frozen
    parsley   cauliflower

Combine ingredients except cauliflower. Simmer uncovered 20 minutes. Add cauliflower and cook until tender-crunchy.

Each portion (⅕ of the recipe) provides: 2 VEG

Zucchini and Carrot Medley   Serves 4

1 pound each carrots and   1 cup water
    zucchini   Salt, coarse pepper

Peel or scrub carrots and cut into ⅛-inch slices. Slice unpared zucchini and set aside. Simmer carrots in water, covered, 10 minutes. Add zucchini and simmer 5 minutes more. Season to taste.

Each portion (¼ of the recipe) provides: 1 VEG

Summer Squash, Turkish-Style   Serves 4

2 yellow squash, sliced   Salt (or garlic salt),
½ cup sliced onion   coarse pepper, to
3 or 4 bay leaves   taste
1 tablespoon lemon juice

Coat a sheet of heavy-duty or double-thick aluminum foil with cooking spray. Mix ingredients together well and arrange on the foil. Close packet and cook on the grill 20 to 25 minutes. Remove bay leaves before serving.

Each portion (¼ of the recipe) provides: 1 VEG

Cheesy Spaghetti Squash

Serves 4

4 cups cooked spaghetti squash	4 tablespoons each grated Parmesan and Romano cheese
4 tablespoons finely chopped fresh parsley	Onion salt and coarse black pepper to taste

Toss ingredients together lightly and serve immediately.

Each portion (¼ of the recipe) provides: 1 PR, 2 VEG

Ratatouille with Eggs

Serves 4

¾ cup bouillon	16-ounce can tomatoes, drained and cut into cubes, or 2 cups of fresh tomatoes, cubed
1 medium red pepper, sliced	
1 medium green pepper, sliced	
1 large onion, sliced	1 teaspoon mixed Italiian herbs
1 clove of garlic, minced	½ teaspoon salt
2 medium or 1 large zucchini, sliced ½-inch thick	Pepper
	3 tablespoons grated Parmesan cheese
1 small eggplant, cut into 1-inch cubes	4 eggs

In a large skillet coated with cooking spray, pour in bouillon, heating slightly. Put in peppers, onion, and garlic; cook until bouillon is almost gone. Add zucchini and eggplant. Cover and cook 20 minutes, stirring occasionally.

Uncover, add tomatoes, herbs, salt, and pepper; cook 10

(continued)

RATATOUILLE WITH EGGS, CONTINUED

more minutes. Sprinkle on cheese. With the back of a spoon, make depressions in the mixture and break an egg into each depression. Cover, cook 5 to 7 more minutes, or until the desired consistency of the egg is reached. Serve immediately.

Each portion (¼ of the recipe) provides: 2 PR, 2 VEG

Grilled Oriental Vegetables   Serves 2

10 ounces frozen mixed Oriental vegetables	¼ teaspoon ground ginger Pinch of fennel seeds (or 5-spice powder)
1 tablespoon light soy sauce	

Coat a sheet of heavy-duty or double-thick foil well with cooking spray. Add the frozen vegetables and remaining ingredients. Wrap tightly. Cook on grill 15 to 20 minutes (or 10 to 12 minutes, if packet has been allowed to thaw).

VARIATION

Grilled Italian Vegetables

Substitute bottled low-calorie Italian seasoned salad dressing for the soy; omit ginger.

Each portion (½ of the recipe) provides: 1 VEG

Vegetable Confetti   Serves 6

½ pound shredded raw carrots	½ pound each julienned zucchini and yellow squash
Small onion, halved, sliced thin	Salt, coarse pepper, to taste
3 tablespoons water (or chicken broth)	

Combine carrots, onion, and water (or chicken broth) in a nonstick skillet which has been coated with cooking spray. Cover and cook 4 to 5 minutes. Stir in remaining ingredients. Cook and stir 1 to 2 minutes, uncovered.

Each portion (⅙ of the recipe) provides: 1 VEG

Vegetable Kebobs

Serves 8

1 medium zucchini, quartered and cut into 1-inch pieces
1 medium yellow squash, quartered and cut into 1-inch pieces
1 red or green bell pepper, seeded and cut into chunks

4 small onions
3 tablespoons light (low-calorie) Italian-style salad dressing
Garlic salt, pepper, to taste

Thread skewers, alternating zucchini, squash, pepper chunks, and whole onions. Brush with salad dressing. Season to taste with garlic salt and pepper. Broil or barbecue 2 inches from heat source for about 8 minutes, turning frequently.

Each portion (⅛ of the recipe) provides: 1 VEG

Golden Apple Sauerkraut

Serves 8

1 yellow (Golden Delicious) apple
1 onion
28-ounce can sauerkraut

2 tablespoons caraway seeds
½ cup white wine (or cider)

Shred the unpared apple by hand or with the shredding disk of a food processor. Chop the onion. Combine them with remaining ingredients. Cover and simmer 1 hour.

Each portion (⅛ of the recipe) provides: 1 VEG

18 Sauces and Marinades

Fu Yung Sauce

Serves 4

1 cup fat-skimmed stock (chicken, turkey, beef, onion, clam broth, etc.)

4 tablespoons dry sherry wine (or additional stock)

3 tablespoons light (sodium-reduced) soy sauce

1 tablespoon cornstarch

¼ teaspoon ground ginger

Optional: 1 clove garlic, minced

Combine ingredients in a saucepan. Cook and stir over moderate heat until mixture simmers, thickens, and clears slightly.

Each portion (¼ of the recipe) provides a small fraction of your PR allowance.

Zesty Salsa

Makes about 2 cups

6 tablespoons minced fresh hot peppers, rinsed or not (or ½ cup diced sweet bell peppers)

1 cup peeled, cubed ripe tomatoes

1 onion, minced

1 or 2 cloves garlic, chopped

5 or 6 tablespoons chopped fresh cilantro leaves (coriander or Mexican parsley

Juice of 1 lime

Salt, pepper, to taste

For the hottest sauce, use whole hot chili peppers, including the seeds. Mince fine, then add to remaining ingredients. However, if you prefer to reduce the heat, use only the pepper part and discard the seeds. To tame the fire even more, chop the chili pepper and rinse it in cold water for several minutes before combining it with the remaining ingredients. For no heat at all, substitute chopped sweet bell pepper.

Combine ingredients and store in the refrigerator. Serve this tasty salsa on anything mild and low-calorie—try it on a baked potato!

> **Each portion (2 tablespoons) provides**
> **a small fraction of your VEG allowance.**

Sauce for Pitaburgers

Makes 1 cup

Good on chicken and fish, too.

½ cup diced (or chopped) cucumber
6 tablespoons plain low-fat yogurt
2 tablespoons each lemon juice and minced fresh (or 2 teaspoons dried) mint or marjoram

Dash each dried oregano, ground nutmeg, and cinnamon
Garlic salt, coarse pepper, to taste

Combine ingredients and refrigerate until serving time.

Serve with broiled or barbecued very lean ground beef round patties that have been basted with lemon juice. Pack each patty into a mini pita pocket with a slice of tomato and a generous amount of sauce.

> **Each portion (¼ cup sauce alone) provides**
> **a small fraction of your VEG and ML allowances.**

Cilantro Sauce   Serves 6

¾ cup undiluted chicken   2 to 4 cloves garlic
    broth, fat-skimmed   ½ teaspoon ground cumin
2 to 3 tablespoons wine   Optional: 1 tablespoon
    vinegar   minced sweet (or hot)
½ cup each fresh cilantro   fresh pepper
    and parsley

Heat broth and vinegar to boiling. Mince remaining ingredients fine and stir in. Or pour hot mixture over remaining ingredients in blender or food processor and process until chopped.

Spoon over baked potatoes, hot drained pasta, plain cooked rice or broiled chicken. To make a sauce for poached seafood, substitute the poaching liquid for the chicken broth.

> Each portion (⅙ of the recipe—sauce alone) provides
> a small fraction of your VEG allowance.

Cucumber Sauce for Seafood   Makes 1 cup

Use instead of high-fat high-salt tartar sauce.

½ cup each shredded (or   2 teaspoons prepared
    chopped) cucumber   mustard
    and light mayonnaise   Coarse pepper (or lemon
2 tablespoons each,   pepper) to taste
    minced fresh dill (or
    parsley) and chives (or
    onion)

Squeeze or press moisture out of cucumber, then combine it with remaining ingredients. Store in refrigerator.

> Limit servings to 1 tablespoon per day.

Meatless Italian Sauce

2 cans (46 ounces each)
    tomato juice
4 tablespoons onion,
    minced
1-pound can of sliced
    mushrooms (or use two
    8-ounce cans)

2 red bell peppers, diced
2 teaspoons sweet basil
2 teaspoons oregano
1 clove garlic, minced
4 beef bouillon cubes

Combine all ingredients in a large, heavy pot. Simmer until thick. You may adjust seasoning for salt and pepper when completed. Use on cooked vegetables or meat.

This sauce freezes well.

Mint Sauce

Serves 4

½ cup each boiling fat-
    skimmed chicken
    broth and minced
    fresh mint leaves
Juice of 1 lemon

1 clove garlic
    Pinch of grated nutmeg
    Salt, coarse pepper, to
    taste

Process ingredients in blender or food processor; toss with hot drained green pasta, cooked brown rice, steamed vegetables, fish or chicken.

VARIATION

Creamy Mint Sauce

Substitute plain low-fat yogurt for the chicken broth. Do not cook the yogurt; simply allow it to warm to room temperature.

> **Each portion (¼ of the recipe—sauce alone) provides a small fraction of your protein allowance.**

Whipped Cottage Cheese

For toppings, dips and other fresh uses, cottage cheese whipped fluffy-smooth in the food processor or blender makes a superior stand-in for sour cream. Its taste and texture are more sour-creamy than yogurt.

Choose a small-curd type of cottage cheese for more tartness, or a mild-flavored large-curd style to vary the flavor. A bit of lemon juice can make it more tangy. Vary the texture by adding a little milk as you process or blend. Add buttermilk for an authentic sour-cream taste. The amount of milk, lemon juice, or buttermilk you add depends on the moisture content of the cottage cheese. Process uncreamed or dry curd cottage cheese with 6 to 8 tablespoons of milk or other liquid. Very wet varieties of cottage cheese may not need any added liquid at all.

Each portion (2½ tablespoons) provides: ½ PR

Lean Cream Sauce Base   Makes 2 cups

⅔ cup plain low-fat yogurt   2 tablespoons instant-
                                         blending flour

Fork-blend ingredients until smooth. Using a wire whisk, gently stir the yogurt mixture into fat-skimmed meat drippings, soups, or the cooking water in which vegetables have been cooked, to thicken and make a sauce. Heat gently, stirring with the whisk, just until heated through and thickened. Season to taste if desired. If sauce is too thick, thin with a little hot water.

Each portion (½ cup of sauce) provides: ⅛ ML, ¼ ST

The next ten sauces provide a variety of interesting meatless toppings for pasta.

Primavera Sauce

Serves 4

1 cup pared, diced
    eggplant
1 cup unpared, sliced
    zucchini
1 onion, sliced
1 green bell pepper,
    seeded, sliced

1 large ripe tomato,
    peeled, cubed
2 cups tomato juice
Optional: 1 clove garlic,
    minced
¼ teaspoon each dried
    thyme and basil

Combine ingredients in a saucepan or skillet. Cover and simmer 10 minutes.

Uncover and continue simmering about 5 minutes, stirring often, until sauce thickens and vegetables are tender but still crisp. (Add a little water if needed.) Spoon immediately over hot drained whole wheat or protein-enriched pasta (allow ½ cup pasta for each serving).

Each portion (¼ of the recipe) provides: 1 VEG
With ½ cup cooked pasta add: 1 ST

Sauce au Jardin

Serves 6

1 cup each fat-skimmed
    chicken broth and
    sliced sweet onion
½ cup each minced celery
    and thinly sliced
    carrots
Optional: garlic, fresh basil,
    and oregano leaves

1 cup each cubed zucchini,
    diced red and green
    bell pepper, and tiny
    cherry tomatoes
¼ cup each minced fresh
    parsley and grated
    Parmesan cheese

Combine chicken broth with onion, celery and carrots. If desired, add garlic, and 1 tablespoon each minced fresh (or

(continued)

SAUCE AU JARDIN, CONTINUED

1 teaspoon each dried) basil and oregano. Cover and simmer 10 minutes. Add zucchini and pepper; simmer 5 minutes more. Add cherry tomatoes and heat through. Spoon over hot drained pasta and sprinkle with parsley and Parmesan.

> **Each portion (⅙ of the recipe) provides: 1½ VEG**
> **With ½ cup cooked pasta add: 1 ST**

Salsa Margarita   Serves 4

3 medium (or 2 large) ripe tomatoes
2 cloves garlic
1 tablespoon olive packing liquid

Salt, coarse pepper, to taste
4 tablespoons chopped fresh basil (or parsley)
½ cup shredded part-skim mozzarella cheese

Peel and dice tomatoes; set aside. Mince garlic and combine with olive liquid in a nonstick pan. Heat garlic until it softens. Stir in tomato and seasonings. Lower heat; warm just until heated through. Spoon over hot drained spaghetti; top with chopped basil and mozzarella.

> **Each portion (¼ of the recipe) provides: 1 PR, ½ VEG**
> **With ½ cup of cooked pasta, add: 1 ST**

Italian Garden Sauce   Serves 6

10-ounce can condensed chicken broth, fat-skimmed
20 ounces frozen mixed Italian-style vegetables
Optional: 1 teaspoon dried oregano

¼ teaspoon grated nutmeg
1½ cups skim milk
2 tablespoons flour
Salt, pepper
4 tablespoons grated Parmesan cheese

In a large nonstick skillet or electric frying pan, heat broth to boiling over high heat. Add vegetables, oregano if you are using it, and nutmeg; simmer uncovered, stirring frequently until nearly all liquid evaporates.

Stir a mixture of the milk and flour into skillet; simmer and stir 3 to 4 minutes, until thickened. Season to taste. Sprinkle with cheese.

> Each portion (⅙ of the recipe) provides: ¼ ML, 1 VEG
> With ½ cup cooked pasta add: 1 ST

Speedy Tomato and Mushroom Sauce   Serves 6

1 cup each
  plain tomato sauce
  dry white wine
  undrained canned stewed
   tomatoes
  mushroom stems and
   pieces

1 teaspoon each dried
   oregano and thyme
Optional: 1 clove garlic,
   minced

Combine ingredients in a saucepan and simmer uncovered 20 to 25 minutes until sauce is reduced and thick. Spoon over pasta.

> Each portion (⅙ of the recipe) provides: 1 VEG
> With ½ cup cooked pasta, add: 1 ST

Basil Sauce   Serves 4

¾ cup boiling water or fat-
   skimmed chicken
   broth
½ cup fresh basil leaves,
   loosely packed

3 cloves garlic
4 tablespoons grated
   Parmesan cheese
Salt, pepper, to taste

Combine ingredients in blender or food processor and process until basil and garlic are minced. Or process by hand,

(continued)

BASIL SAUCE, CONTINUED

using a mortar and pestle to mash basil and garlic together,
then mix with remaining ingredients.

Add the sauce to hot drained pasta and toss lightly.

> **Each portion (¼ of the recipe) provides a small fraction of
> your protein allowance.**
>
> **With ½ cup cooked pasta, add: 1 ST**

Pesto Sauce   Serves 6

2 cups pot-style low-fat
    cottage (or skim milk
    ricotta) cheese
2 large cloves garlic,
    peeled
1 cup each, loosely packed
    fresh parsley and basil
    (or raw spinach)

1 cup boiling water
10 tablespoons grated
    Parmesan (or
    Romano) cheese
Salt, coarse pepper, to
    taste
3 cups tender-cooked
    spaghetti

Have cheese at room temperature. Combine with remaining ingredients, except spaghetti, in blender (or food processor, using steel blade). Cover; blend smooth. Toss with
hot drained spaghetti.

> **Each portion (⅙ of the recipe, including pasta)
> provides: 2 PR, 1 ST**

Spinach Ricotta Sauce   Serves 6

1 cup part-skim ricotta
    cheese
1 clove garlic

1 cup raw spinach leaves
Grated nutmeg, lemon
    peel, salt, pepper

Have ricotta at room temperature. Combine with garlic and
spinach in food processor, using the steel blade. Process

completely smooth; season to taste. Toss with hot drained pasta.

> **Each portion (⅙ of the recipe) provides: 1 PR, ⅓ VEG**
> **With ½ cup cooked pasta add: 1 ST**

Italian Pepper Sauce
Serves 4

1 tablespoon olive packing liquid	3 green (or red) sweet peppers, diced or shredded
1 onion, minced	
1 clove garlic, minced	2 tablespoons each minced fresh basil and parsley
1 cup fat-skimmed chicken broth	Optional: Salt, coarse pepper, to taste

Coat a nonstick skillet with cooking spray. Add olive liquid, onion and garlic; cook and stir 2 minutes. Add remaining ingredients; cover and simmer 7 to 8 minutes. Toss with hot drained pasta.

> **Each portion (¼ of the recipe) provides: 1 VEG**
> **With ½ cup cooked pasta, add: 1 ST**

Piedmont Parsley Sauce
Serves 4

1 cup fat-skimmed hot chicken broth	3 tablespoons minced fresh basil leaves
1 to 2 tablespoons lemon juice (or vinegar)	2 cloves garlic
1 cup chopped fresh Italian parsley	1 anchovy, chopped (or 1 tablespoon Worcestershire sauce)
	Coarse pepper to taste

Combine liquid ingredients and heat to boiling. Chop remaining ingredients by hand and add to hot sauce.

(continued)

PIEDMONT PARSLEY SAUCE, CONTINUED

Or combine all ingredients in blender or food processor and chop coarsely with on-off pulse setting.

Pour over hot drained pasta and toss together.

> Each portion (¼ of the recipe) provides a small fraction of your protein requirement.
>
> With ½ cup cooked pasta, add: 1 ST

Baste à la Grecque   Makes about ¾ cup

6 or 8 tablespoons plain
    low-fat yogurt
Juice of 1 lemon
3 tablespoons chopped
    fresh (or 1 tablespoon
    dried) mint

2 teaspoons fresh (or ½
    teaspoon dried)
    oregano
Pinch each grated
    nutmeg and cinnamon
Salt (or garlic salt),
    pepper, to taste

Fold ingredients together. Spread over lean lamb steaks, hamburger, chicken, or fish. Refrigerate until cooking time. Broil or barbecue to desired doneness.

> Each portion (2 tablespoons) provides a small fraction of your protein allowance.

Chinese Barbecue Sauce   Makes about ¾ cup

¾ cup soy sauce
2 to 3 packets low-calorie
    sweetener

1 tablespoon grated orange
    rind
1 clove of garlic, minced
Pepper to taste

Mix ingredients. Marinate any meat you wish for 1 hour or overnight. Prepare as desired.

> Nutrients provided by this sauce are negligible.

Marinade for Meat or Poultry   Makes about ½ cup

1½ teaspoons dry mustard	⅛ teaspoon garlic powder
¾ teaspoon ground ginger	6 tablespoons soy sauce
Pepper to taste	3 tablespoons lemon juice

Mix ingredients well. Marinate for 1 hour or overnight. Prepare meat as desired.

Nutrients provided by this marinade are negligible.

Tangy Marinade   Serves 2

½ cup plain low-fat yogurt	1 teaspoon dried herbs
1 tablespoon each	(thyme, oregano,
prepared mustard,	savory, rosemary, etc.)
Worcestershire sauce,	Salt (or seasoned salt),
and lemon juice	coarse black pepper, to
1 clove garlic, minced	taste

Combine ingredients and spread over lean beef top-round steak, flank steak, or cut-up frying chicken pieces. Cover and marinate 30 minutes at room temperature or several hours in the refrigerator. Leaving the mixture on the food, broil or barbecue until done.

Each portion (½ of the recipe) provides: ⅓ ML

Spicy Cajun Marinade   Makes about 1 cup

¾ cup spicy tomato juice	2 cloves garlic, minced
3 tablespoons each	½ teaspoon (dried) thyme
Worcestershire sauce	Optional: 1 to 2 teaspoons
and lemon juice	hot sauce

Combine ingredients. Marinate meat or poultry for about 30 minutes at room temperature, or for several hours in the

(continued)

refrigerator. Marinate fish for a shorter period, depending upon type and thickness.

Nutrients provided by this marinade are negligible.

Hawaiian Marinade   Makes about 1¼ cups

½ cup each white wine,   2 cloves garlic, minced
    unsweetened   1 tablespoon ground
    pineapple juice   ginger
 3 tablespoons soy sauce

Combine ingredients. Pour over meat or poultry and refrigerate several hours. If meat is frozen, put it in a plastic bag and add marinating liquid. Let meat defrost in mixture.

Nutrients provided by this marinade are negligible.

19 Snacks, Drinks, and Desserts

Yogurt Cheese

Makes about 1 cup

Drip-type coffee cone and
    filter paper

Optional: pinch of salt
2 cups plain low-fat yogurt

Line a coffee cone with filter paper and arrange it over a coffee pot. If you are using salt, gently mix into the yogurt and empty the yogurt into the lined coffee cone. Put everything in the refrigerator and allow the yogurt to drain 6 to 8 hours until reduced by half (more or less, for a firmer or softer cheese).

Cheese may be wrapped in the filter paper. The drained liquid is known as "whey" and is very nutritious though low in calories; save it to add to soups or stews.

Each portion (2½ tablespoons) provides: 1 PR

VARIATION

Pimiento and Olive Cheese

Makes 1¼ cups

1 cup Yogurt Cheese made
    without added salt
¼ cup stuffed Spanish-style
    green olives, minced

1 tablespoon olive brine
    (from jar of olives)

Mix ingredients lightly. Spoon into a crock, cover and store in the refrigerator.

Each portion (2½ tablespoons) provides: 1 PR

Hungarian Chive Cheese   Makes about 1 cup

This recipe is a bit like Liptauer cheese, without the excess calories—and without the anchovies.

1 cup Yogurt Cheese (see page 201)	2 teaspoons each chopped chives (or onions), caraway seeds, prepared mustard, and drained capers Paprika

Gently mix Yogurt Cheese with remaining ingredients, except paprika. Shape into a mound and cover all over with paprika. Serve with crackers or bell pepper scoops.

Each portion (2¼ tablespoons) provides: 1 PR

Iced Coffee, Jamaican-Style   Serves 4

4 cups fresh strong coffee   Dash of ground allspice
2 teaspoons rum flavoring

Combine coffee, rum flavoring and allspice; chill. Pour over ice cubes in 4 tall glasses.

Nutrients provided by this beverage are negligible.

Light Wine Cooler   Serves 1

Dry red or white wine   lemon-lime soda, or plain
Sugar-free fruit or diet   seltzer

Put 5 ounces red or white wine in a tall glass over ice; fill with soda and stir.

Limit to one serving a day as the allowance for alcoholic beverage.

Zesty Tomato Cooler   Serves 1

¾ cup tomato juice
1 tablespoon lemon juice

Dash each Worces-
     tershire and hot pepper
     sauce
Optional: 1 celery stalk

Combine juices and flavorings; pour over ice cubes in a tall glass. Use celery stalk as stirrer, if desired.

Each portion (1 cooler) provides: 1 VEG

3-Juice Fruit Punch   Makes 14 6-ounce servings

6 ounces each unsweetened
     orange, grape, and
     pineapple frozen juice
     concentrates

3 quarts club soda
Optional: fresh fruit for
     garnish

Allow fruit juice concentrates to thaw; combine with soda over a block of ice in a large punch bowl. Garnish with fresh fruit, if desired.

For single servings: Combine the 3 thawed juice concentrates in a pitcher and store in the refrigerator. To make 1 drink, pour 2 or 3 tablespoons of the "syrup" over ice in a tall glass, then fill to the top with sparkling water.

Each portion (6 ounces) provides: 1 FR

Juicy Cooler   Serves 1

Frozen orange juice
     concentrate
Bottled white grape juice

Brandy extract
Club soda

Store the thawed undiluted orange juice concentrate and bottled grape juice in the refrigerator. Combine 2 table-

(continued)

spoons orange juice concentrate, 4 tablespoons white grape juice, and a few drops of brandy extract with club soda in a tall glass over ice.

VARIATION

Use red grape juice, rum extract.

                              Each portion (1 cooler) provides: 1 FR

Chomocha Milkshake   Serves 1

1 tablespoon plain cocoa	5 tablespoons dry skim
1 teaspoon instant coffee	milk powder
½ cup boiling water	1 or 2 packets low-calorie
1 cup ice cubes	sweetener
	Few drops vanilla extract

Combine cocoa, coffee, and boiling water in blender; cover and process until dissolved. Fill a 1-cup measure with ice cubes. Add to the blender along with the remaining ingredients and process until ice is completely dissolved and shake is thick and frothy. Fills a large glass.

                        Each portion (1 milkshake) provides: 1 ML

Mousse Napoleon   Serves 4

2 envelopes plain gelatin	1 cup fresh skim milk
4 tablespoons cold water	1 package (4-serving)
1 cup hot coffee	vanilla instant pudding
2 teaspoons brandy extract	mix
2 cups part-skim ricotta	1 tablespoon plain cocoa
cheese	powder

Combine gelatin and cold water in blender or food processor. Wait 1 minute for gelatin to soften. Meanwhile, combine coffee and brandy extract; heat to boiling. Add to blender; cover and process until all gelatin granules are dissolved. Add ricotta and process until completely smooth and nongrainy. Add milk and pudding mix; process smooth. Spoon most of the mixture into shallow bowl, reserving half a cup. Combine the reserved half cup with cocoa and mix well. Spoon the cocoa mixture in stripes on top of the dessert. Then use the tip of a knife to draw through the stripes in the opposite direction, making a Napoleon-type swirl pattern. Or for a marbled mousse, simply drizzle the chocolate mixture into the dessert and swirl lightly (don't overmix). Chill several hours until set.

Each portion (¼ of the recipe) provides: 1 PR, ½ ST, ½ ML

No-Cook Chocolate Mousse   Serves 4

1 large egg	½ cup low-fat cottage
1 envelope plain gelatin	cheese
1 tablespoon cornstarch	½ cup cold, low-fat milk
1 tablespoon cold water	2½ tablespoons plain cocoa
1 cup boiling water	9 packets low-calorie
1 teaspoon instant coffee	sweetener

Combine egg, gelatin, cornstarch, and cold water in a blender container. Blend just until gelatin and cornstarch are moist. Wait 1 minute for gelatin granules to soften, then add boiling water. Cover and blend.

Add remaining ingredients, except the sweetener. Blend until mixture is completely smooth and free of granules. Add the sweetener and blend. Pour into 4 dessert dishes and let set.

Each portion (¼ of the recipe) provides: 1 PR

Fruit Mousse Medley   Serves 8

6-ounce can orange juice concentrate

2 eggs, separated

8-ounce can juice-packed pineapple rings

Water

1 envelope plain gelatin

¾ cup part-skim ricotta cheese

Optional: low-calorie sweetener to equal 10 teaspoons (5 packets)

Pinch of salt

1 eating orange, pared, cut in wedges

1 banana, sliced vertically

Thaw orange juice concentrate but don't dilute. Separate eggs; put whites in an electric mixer bowl and yolks in blender or food processor.

Drain pineapple and reserve juice. Add water to pineapple juice to make ½ cup; combine in a saucepan with gelatin. Wait 1 minute, then heat gently until gelatin melts. Remove from heat.

Beat egg yolks in food processor or blender, then add pineapple juice-gelatin mixture through the small opening while motor runs. Add undiluted orange juice concentrate, ricotta, and low-calorie sweetener, if desired. Cover and process until completely smooth and blended. Chill until partly set.

Add a pinch of salt to egg whites and beat until stiff peaks form. Gently but thoroughly fold partly set gelatin mixture into beaten egg whites.

Arrange pineapple rings, orange wedges, and banana slices vertically inside a glass casserole; press lightly to the sides. Spoon in gelatin mixture. Chill in refrigerator until set.

Each portion (⅛ of the recipe) provides: ⅛ PR, 1½ FR

Orange Cheese Mousse   Serves 10

4 tablespoons orange juice, divided	4 single-serving packets sugar-free vanilla milkshake mix
1 cup boiling water	
1 tablespoon plain gelatin	Optional: 1 pint fresh strawberries, sliced
12 ounces cottage cheese	

Heat 2 tablespoons juice with water until boiling. Meanwhile, combine remaining 2 tablespoons juice with gelatin in blender or food processor. Allow gelatin to soften 1 minute. Add boiling water mixture to gelatin. Process until gelatin granules are dissolved; use a rubber scraper on the side of the container and process again. Add cottage cheese and process until completely smooth and creamy. Add vanilla mix and process completely smooth.

Chill until set. Arrange sliced strawberries (or other fresh fruit) on top of mousse before serving, if desired.

VARIATION

Orange Chocolate Cheese Mousse

Substitute sugar-free chocolate milkshake mix for the vanilla mix. Top with fresh orange slices, if desired.

Each portion (¹⁄₁₀ of the recipe) provides: ⅓ PR. ⅓ ML
With fruit add: ½ FR

Lime Mousse   Serves 6

2 eggs	1 cup ice cubes
1 envelope plain gelatin	5 packages sugar-free vanilla milkshake mix
1 cup boiling water	
½ cup fresh lime juice	

Beat eggs and gelatin together. Wait 1 minute until gelatin softens, then beat in boiling water, until gelatin granules
(continued)

LIME MOUSSE, CONTINUED

melt. Add lime juice. Beat in ice cubes, one at a time. Beat
in milkshake mix. Spoon into dessert dishes and chill until
set.

Each portion (⅙ of the recipe) provides: ¾ ML

Peach Cheesecake   Serves 12

1 envelope plain gelatin	Optional: 6 packets low-
¾ cup unsweetened peach	calorie sweetener
nectar (or other fruit	4 large graham crackers,
juice), divided	broken up
8 ounces low-fat cream	1½ cups fresh sliced
cheese (or	peaches (or apricots)
Neufchâtel)	
8 ounces uncreamed	
cottage cheese	

Spray a nonstick square cake pan generously with cooking
spray. Combine gelatin and 2 tablespoons peach nectar in
blender or food processor. While gelatin softens, heat remaining peach nectar to boiling. Add hot nectar to gelatin
mixture; cover and process until gelatin granules are completely dissolved. Add cream cheese, cottage cheese, and
sweetener, if used; process completely smooth. Arrange
graham crackers in the bottom of the cake pan. Spoon
cheese mixture over crackers and chill until set. Just before
serving, peel and slice peaches (coat peach slices with
lemon juice and sweetener to taste, if desired) and arrange
slices on top of cheese filling. Cut into squares to serve.

Each portion (1/12 of the recipe) provides: 1 PR, ⅙ ST, ¼ FR

Fruited Cheesecake   Serves 6

4 eggs, separated
1½ cups low-fat cottage
    cheese
4 tablespoons plain or
    vanilla low-fat yogurt

7 to 9 packets low-calorie
    sweetener, divided
3 cups sliced fresh
    strawberries, or a
    mixture of fresh fruit
2 tablespoons lemon juice

Separate egg yolks into a blender and egg whites into a mixing bowl. Add cheese and yogurt to the egg yolks. Cover and blend until smooth.

Beat egg whites stiff with electric mixer. Pour egg yolk-cheese mixture into egg whites and gently, but thoroughly, fold together (don't overmix).

Spray an 8- or 9-inch springform pan, then spoon batter into it. Bake in a preheated 350-degree oven for approximately 45 minutes, until puffy. Remove cake from the oven and let it set for 10 minutes. Sprinkle with 3 packets of sweetener. When cool, chill in refrigerator.

While cake is chilling, stir the fruit together with the lemon juice and the remaining sweetener. Refrigerate until serving time. Spoon fruit onto the cheesecake just before serving. (Note: Canned fruit, drained, may be used instead of fresh fruit.)

Each portion (⅙ of the recipe) provides: 1 PR, 1 FR

Crustless Cherry Cheese Pie   Serves 10

1 envelope plain gelatin
1 egg
4 tablespoons apple juice
¾ cup boiling water

12-ounces low-fat pot-style
    cottage cheese
8 packets low-calorie
    sweetener
1 cup fresh cherries

Combine gelatin and egg in blender or food processor; process until mixed. Combine juice and water; heat to boiling.

(continued)

CRUSTLESS CHERRY CHEESE PIE, CONTINUED

With machine running, add hot liquid through the opening
in top. Process until gelatin granules are dissolved. Stop
machine and scrape down the container sides with a rubber
scraper, then process again. Add cottage cheese and sweetener; process until cheese is smooth. Chill until mixture
begins to set.

Meanwhile, cut cherries in half and remove pits. Fold
gently into cheese mixture, then spoon filling into a glass
pie dish.

Each portion (1/10 of the recipe) provides: 1 PR, ½ FR

Apricot Cheese Pie   Serves 8

1 tablespoon diet   3 eggs
   margarine   Pinch of salt
½ cup graham cracker   ½ cup each golden raisins
   crumbs   and finely chopped
1 pound low-fat pot-style   dried apricot halves
   cottage cheese   Ground cinnamon
¼ cup apricot nectar

Spread margarine over bottom of a nonstick 8-inch pie pan.
Sprinkle on graham cracker crumbs; press firmly over bottom of pan.

Combine cheese, nectar, eggs, and salt in blender or food
processor container. Process smooth, scraping down sides
of container with rubber scraper. Pour half of this filling
mixture into pie pan. Sprinkle raisins and apricots evenly
over filling. Pour on remaining filling covering all fruit.
Sprinkle with cinnamon.

Bake in preheated 325-degree oven 45 to 55 minutes, or
until filling is set. Cool before serving.

Each portion (⅛ of the pie) provides: 1 PR, ½ ST, 1 FR

Black and White Pie   Serves 6

1 cup low-fat milk (divided)	8 packets low-calorie sweetener, divided
1 envelope plain gelatin	4 tablespoons plain cocoa powder
¾ cup low-fat cottage cheese	2 egg whites
2 teaspoons vanilla extract or rum flavoring	Pinch of salt

Put half the milk into a saucepan. Sprinkle the gelatin over it. Soften 1 minute, then heat gently, stirring until the gelatin is completely dissolved.

Place cottage cheese in blender. Cover and blend until completely smooth. Add gelatin mixture, remaining milk and vanilla. Cover and blend until smooth. Put half of the blended mixture into a mixing bowl and set it aside.

To the half of the mixture remaining in the blender, add 4 packets sweetener and cocoa. Blend thoroughly. Pour into a sprayed, 8-inch pie pan and chill until partially set—about 30 minutes.

Beat egg whites and salt until stiff. Gradually beat in the remaining sweetener. Gently but thoroughly fold into the vanilla half of the mixture. Spoon over chocolate layer and chill several hours until completely set.

Each portion (⅙ of the pie) provides: 1 PR

Crustless Chocolate Cinnamon Pie   Serves 8

1 cup cold skim milk,   1 package (4-serving)
    divided   sugar-free instant
1 envelope plain gelatin   chocolate pudding mix
¾ cup boiling water   1 teaspoon vanilla extract
4 or 5 ice cubes   ½ teaspoon ground
8 ounces pot-style low-fat   cinnamon
    cottage cheese   Optional: 2 or 3 packets
                                    low-calorie sweetener

Put 3 or 4 tablespoons of milk in the bottom of food processor or blender container and sprinkle with gelatin. Wait 1 minute until gelatin is soft, then add boiling water. Process until gelatin is completely dissolved (scrape sides of container with rubber scraper). Add ice cubes; process until melted. Add cottage cheese; process until completely smooth and creamy. Add remaining ingredients; process smooth (add sweetener to taste last, if desired). Spoon the mixture into a glass pie dish.

Each portion (⅛ of the recipe) provides: ½ PR, ½ ST, ⅛ ML

Crustless Chomocha Pie   Serves 8

1 envelope plain gelatin   1 cup each fresh skim milk
6 tablespoons water   and part-skim ricotta
2 teaspoons instant coffee   cheese
    powder   4-serving package sugar-
                                    free instant chocolate
                                    pudding mix

Sprinkle gelatin on water. Wait 1 minute, then heat gently, until gelatin dissolves. Remove from heat and stir in instant coffee until dissolved.

In food processor or blender, combine milk and ricotta; process completely smooth. Add gelatin mixture; process smooth. Add pudding mix; process smooth. Chill several hours in glass pie plate and keep refrigerated. (Leftover pie can be sliced into single-serving wedges and frozen. Thaw several hours in the refrigerator before serving.)

Each portion (⅛ of the recipe) provides: ½ PR, ½ ST

Poached Pears with Raspberry Sauce   Serves 12

This recipe comes from Adrian's Café in Philadelphia.

2 quarts water	6 to 8 ounces frozen
Half lemon, sliced	unsweetened
1 cinnamon stick	raspberries
6 firm fresh pears	Low-calorie sweetener
	Optional: fresh mint leaves

Fill a pot with cold water and add lemon slices and cinnamon stick.

Peel the pears, leaving the stem and a little cap of skin near the stem. Place each pear in the cold water as soon as it's peeled. Simmer just until cooked through but not mushy, about 6 to 8 minutes. Drain pears on paper towels, then chill thoroughly in the refrigerator. Split each pear in half and remove the core with a tablespoon.

To make sauce, thaw the raspberries and puree them smooth in the blender or food processor, sweetening to taste. Arrange each cored pear half on top of its sauce. Garnish with some fresh mint, if desired.

Each portion (1/12 of the recipe) provides: 1½ FR

Blueberry Jel-Low   Serves 4

1 envelope plain gelatin
1 cup each cold water,
    chilled bottled
    unsweetened grape
    juice

6 packets low-calorie
    sweetener, or to taste
1 pint fresh blueberries

Sprinkle gelatin on ½ cup water in a small saucepan. Wait
1 minute, then heat gently until melted. Remove from heat
and stir in remaining half-cup water, grape juice and
sweetener. Refrigerate until syrupy, then fold in berries.
Chill until set.

Each portion (¼ of the recipe) provides: 1 FR

Luscious Lime Parfait   Serves 10

1 envelope unflavored
    gelatin
¼ cup cold water
1 cup boiling water
½ cup low-fat cottage
    cheese

⅓ cup lime juice
3 egg whites
Pinch of salt
8 packets low-calorie
    sweetener

Sprinkle gelatin over cold water in blender. Wait 1 minute
for gelatin to soften, then add boiling water. Blend until
gelatin is dissolved. Add cottage cheese and blend until
smooth. Add lime juice and blend. Refrigerate until partially set.

Beat egg whites and salt until soft peaks form. Beat in
sweetener.

Beat partially set gelatin mixture until light and fluffy.
Gently fold into beaten egg whites. Spoon into 10 parfait
glasses. Top each with a sprinkle of grated peel or a few
graham cracker crumbs, if desired.

Each portion (¹⁄₁₀ of the recipe) provides: ½ PR

Frozen Bananas

Bananas are easy to freeze and have lots of uses in the low-cal sugar-free kitchen: in drinks, for ice cream and frozen yogurts, in parfaits.

Simply peel and slice them thick or thin. Spread the slices in a single layer, touching, on a sheet of plastic or foil and cover tightly to keep out the air. Label and freeze, then take out only what you need.

The best bananas for freezing are the ripest, skins generously freckled. The riper they are, the more natural sweetness. Storing banana slices in the freezer for later use is a very good way to use up overripe bananas that have lots of flavor but are too mushy for out-of-hand eating. However, for best color, taste, and texture, frozen bananas should be used fairly soon, within a few weeks if possible. If you plan to freeze them longer, squirt some lemon juice over the slices before you wrap and freeze them. Lemon adds delicious tang to these recipes; you might like the lemon-kissed versions better.

Banana "Ice Cream"   Serves 4

3 small (or 2 large) ripe   6 or 7 tablespoons fresh
   bananas, peeled, sliced,   skim milk
   and frozen

Put the frozen banana slices in your food processor (using the steel blade) or in a blender. Process until frozen bananas are chopped and grainy but still frozen. Add the milk a few tablespoons at a time and process until smooth and creamy, the texture of frozen custard. Serve immediately. Don't add too much milk or process too long or mixture will become too soft.

With an electric mixer: If you don't have a food processor

(continued)

BANANA "ICE CREAM," CONTINUED

or blender, you can make Banana "Ice Cream" with an electric mixer. However, it won't be as quick and convenient. Here's how: Don't freeze the bananas. Peel them and combine them with the milk in an electric mixer bowl, then beat them smooth. Spoon the mixture into ice cube trays and freeze firm. Remove banana cubes from freezer and put them in the electric mixer bowl. Let soften slightly several minutes, then quickly beat the cubes into a fluffy frost that resembles frozen custard. Serve immediately.

If you have an ice cream maker, beat the fresh banana and milk together, then spoon the mixture into the appliance and process according to manufacturer's directions.

VARIATIONS

Frozen Banana Yogurt

Substitute plain low-fat yogurt for the milk.

Each portion (¼ of the recipe) provides: 1 FR, ⅛ ML

Orange Banana Sherbet

Substitute orange juice for the milk.

Provides 1⅛ FR

Other Variations

Sweeten to taste, if desired, with 1 or 2 packets low-calorie sweetener. Make a tangy banana-buttermilk sorbet by using buttermilk instead of milk. Use other fruit juices: pineapple, apple, or apricot, or try grape for a frozen Banana Blush. Vary the flavor with a few drops of brandy or rum flavoring, or use 2 tablespoons rum and 4 or 5 tablespoons water instead of milk. Flavor with vanilla or coconut extract, if desired.

Banana Strawberry Sundae   Serves 4

Better than a banana split!

Banana Ice Cream (see   1 cup fresh (or thawed)
   page 215)   unsweetened
                                    strawberries

Make Banana Ice Cream as directed and spoon into 3
stemmed goblets or sundae dishes. Store the desserts
briefly in the freezer while you prepare the sauce.

Rinse, but do not wash, food processor or blender. Put
the washed hulled strawberries (or thawed strawberries)
into the unit and process until chopped or pureed into a
bright red sauce (sweeten, if desired, with a few packets
low-calorie sweetener. Drizzle the sauce over the ice cream.

Each portion (¼ of the recipe) provides: 1¼ FR, ⅛ ML

Bananectarina "Ice Cream"   Serves 5

2 bananas, peeled, sliced   1 large unpeeled tree-ripe
   thin, and frozen (see p.   nectarine (or 2 small
   215)   unpeeled peaches,
                                    sliced)
                              2 tablespoons ice-cold
                               water

Slice the bananas thin and freeze. At dessert time, dice the
nectarine (no need to peel, the flecks of peel add color,
flavor, and fiber). Combine ingredients in food processor
and process smooth, adding another tablespoon or two of
water, if needed.

Each portion (⅕ of the recipe) provides: 1 FR

Berry Banana "Ice Cream"   Serves 6

This recipe is high in fiber.

½ pint raspberries (or   2 bananas, peeled, sliced
   blackberries)   thin, and frozen (see p.
3 or 4 tablespoons water   215)

Rinse raspberries and reserve some for garnish. Combine
raspberries and frozen banana slices in food processor; process into soft-serve ice creamlike texture, adding water a
tablespoon at a time. (If you are not milk-intolerant, you
could substitute skim milk for the water.) Serve immediately, garnished with a few fresh berries. (For a sweeter
dessert add low-calorie sweetener to taste.)

VARIATION

Banana Strawberry "Ice Cream"

Substitute sliced fresh strawberries for the raspberries.

Each portion (⅙ of the recipe) provides: 1 FR

Banana Pineapple Sundae   Serves 5

2 bananas, peeled, sliced   Few drops rum flavoring
   thin, and frozen (see p.   4 tablespoons juice-packed
215)   crushed pineapple,
2 to 4 tablespoons   drained
   unsweetened pineapple
juice

Combine frozen bananas with juice and rum flavoring in
food processor. Process until the texture of soft-serve ice
cream. Serve immediately in parfait glasses with crushed
pineapple on top.

Each portion (⅕ of the recipe) provides: 1 FR

Tricolor Banana Parfaits

Serves 6

2 ripe bananas, peeled, sliced thin, and frozen (see p. 215)

1 cup each fresh blueberries and sliced strawberries

To assemble parfaits, arrange the banana slices between a layer of blueberries and a layer of strawberries in a tulip sundae bowl.

Each portion (⅙ of the recipe) provides: 1½ FR

Frozen Banana Milkshake

Serves 1

One of the best ways to use frozen banana slices is in frosty milkshakes. The banana chills the milk.

Several slices frozen banana (equal to half a banana) (see p. 215)

6 ounces fresh skim milk
Few drops vanilla extract

Combine in blender and process smooth. Add a shake of cinnamon, if desired.

Each portion (1 shake) provides: ¾ ML, 1 FR

Index